Take Your *Back* Back

Take Your *Back* Back

Whole Health Healing for Low Back Pain

Christine Goertz, DC, PhD

Simon Element

New York Amsterdam/Antwerp London
Toronto Sydney/Melbourne New Delhi

SIMON ELEMENT

An Imprint of Simon & Schuster, LLC
1230 Avenue of the Americas
New York, NY 10020

This publication contains the opinions and ideas of its author. It is intended to provide helpful and informative material on the subjects addressed in the publication. It is sold with the understanding that the author and publisher are not engaged in rendering medical, health, or any other kind of personal professional services in the book. Readers should consult a medical, health or other competent professional before adopting any of the suggestions in this book or drawing inferences from it.

The author and publisher specifically disclaim all responsibility for any liability, loss or risk, personal or otherwise, which is incurred as a consequence, directly or indirectly, of the use and application of any of the contents of this book.

The authorized representative in the EEA is Simon & Schuster Nederland B.V., Herculesplein 96, 3584 AA Utrecht, Netherlands. info@simonandschuster.nl

First Simon Element trade paperback edition October 2026

SIMON ELEMENT and colophon are registered trademarks of Simon & Schuster, LLC

Interior design by Julia Jacintho

Manufactured in the United States of America

1 3 5 7 9 10 8 6 4 2

Library of Congress Cataloging-in-Publication Data has been applied for.

ISBN 978-1-6682-1163-2
ISBN 978-1-6682-1164-9 (ebook)

This book is dedicated to the more than 600 million people worldwide living with low back pain each year and to my husband, Randy DeGeest, whose unwavering love and support made writing this book possible.

Contents

Introduction

If you are reading this book, it's likely that you or someone close to you has low back pain. You are not alone. About 85 percent of people experience low back pain at some point in their lives, and it affects more than 600 million people every year. It is the number one cause of disability in the world and one of the most common reasons people visit a primary care physician in the United States. Billions of dollars are spent on treatments, more than is spent on almost any other condition or disease, often on approaches that fail to deliver the desired results.

If your low back pain is new, you may be frightened by how much it hurts and worry that something life-threatening is causing it. If you have had low back pain for a while, you may feel hopeless and believe that the pain will never go away, no matter what you do. I can relate. When I had low back pain in my late twenties, I felt this way.

If I had low back pain when I started the drive home from school that day, I don't remember it. However, I vividly recall that the pain was so bad I could barely make it out of the car once I reached my driveway. When the pain was still there the following morning, my first instinct was to see a chiropractor. After all, I was a first-year chiropractic student. Although the X-rays they took at the student clinic showed nothing concerning, and

I felt better right after receiving spinal manipulation, the pain returned by dinnertime. This cycle repeated over several visits during the next ten days with no overall change in my condition. I stopped going and doubts about a career in chiropractic crept into my mind. I was drawn to the profession by its whole-person, natural approach to care, but this was my first experience as a patient.

My next strategy was to power through the pain on my own. I took over-the-counter Advil several times a day and spent every moment possible in the only position that alleviated the pain: lying flat on the floor with my knees bent. I gritted my teeth through the pain to attend class, prepare meals, and take my child to preschool.

About four months into my low back pain experience, I was sitting in biochemistry class when suddenly the pain became unbearable. The pain was the same, but my ability to tolerate it suddenly changed. I stopped listening to the professor and instead focused inwardly on the emotions tumbling over one another in my head. Fear that the pain would never go away or might get even worse. Anger and then despair over my increasing inability to enjoy life's most basic activities. All I wanted was to make dinner, play with my son, or learn from a lecture.

Then I had a horrible thought. What if something was terribly wrong? Maybe I needed surgery. I thought about the fifteen pounds I had recently lost. Oh my God, did I have cancer? As soon as class ended, I made the first available appointment with a medical physician.

When I showed up a week later in close to a state of panic, my primary care physician asked me a few questions. Had I noticed any changes, such as complete bowel or bladder control loss, since my pain started? Was I experiencing increasing weakness or numbness in my legs? Did I have a fever, pain, or burning sensation while urinating? Did the pain wake me up at night? No, no, no, and no. "You don't have cancer," she finally said in response to the first question I had asked her. "Or anything else that I can find." She did not look me in the eyes again as she prescribed a higher dose of Advil than what was available over the counter and wrote "provided supportive care" in my healthcare record. The pills helped take the edge off the pain at times but did not make a meaningful difference in my ability to function normally. I did not feel supported.

Almost a year passed with little change in my condition. I confessed to a fellow student that I had decided to leave chiropractic school. I was in too much pain every day to focus on my studies. More importantly, I had become convinced that chiropractic "didn't work."

That fellow student's response was to convince me to see her chiropractor. Dr. David listened carefully to my story and asked the same questions the medical physician had about my pain. However, he also asked a few new ones. For instance, could I remember doing anything unusual in the day or so before my pain started?

A forgotten memory popped into my head. That morning so long ago, my eighteen-month-old son had a well-child visit with his pediatrician and fell asleep in the car on the way back to day care. I decided to carry him in his car seat, a combined weight of about forty pounds, into day care so that he could continue to sleep a little longer. When we got there, I set the car seat on the ground and then twisted to pick him up while holding the heavy industrial door open with one foot. I felt a twinge in my low back at the time, but it was so mild I never thought to connect this experience with my pain later that day.

Dr. David also asked about other aspects of my life. Was I sleeping well? Did I feel depressed or anxious? When he learned that I was experiencing high levels of stress and anxiety, he reassured me that these feelings were widespread in people with chronic low back pain. His diagnosis was that I had injured a disc in my low back when picking up my son in his car seat. He was also concerned that I was suffering from an anxiety disorder.

I had been struggling with my low back pain for so long, mostly all by myself, feeling as if others believed it was "all in my head." As Dr. David spoke, I felt heard for the first time in many months. He validated that something "real" was wrong with me and gave me hope that help was available. His treatment plan had several components. He used a type of spinal manipulation on me that I had not heard of before, called flexion distraction. He suggested that I start walking, going a little farther each day, and gave me some low back exercises to do at home. He also recommended I consider seeing a psychologist to help with my anxiety. I saw Dr. David six times in two weeks, followed by about six more visits over the next two months.

As recommended, I also made an appointment with Dr. Jeff, a clinical psychologist. I told him that thoughts about my pain were a constant companion, and I was now convinced I would be disabled for the rest of my life. The pain and anxiety made it difficult for me to be present for my active toddler. I told him my coursework was too demanding given my current level of pain and I was seriously considering leaving chiropractic college. I felt trapped by my substantial student loan debt and lacked a clear alternative life plan. Voicing these feelings out loud for the first time brought profound relief that grew into calm during several sessions over the next few weeks. Dr. Jeff used a psychological therapy approach called cognitive behavioral therapy (CBT) with me. The purpose of CBT is to help people change their thoughts and, even more importantly, their behaviors. The techniques I learned helped me stop worrying so much about, well, everything. He also recommended meditation to help with my stress and taught me a basic box breathing technique. What I learned from him would become lifelong practices. Within six weeks, my pain was 80 percent gone. After three months, I was no longer experiencing daily pain.

My experience left me with more questions than answers. What causes low back pain? Why does it sometimes hurt for so long? What treatments work best and why? For example, how was Dr. David able to help me so much when my first chiropractic experience did not help at all? I set out to find the answers to these questions. I graduated from Northwestern Health Sciences University. I got my PhD from the University of Minnesota. I worked at the National Institutes of Health. I led the largest chiropractic research center in the United States. Now I am a professor at Duke University School of Medicine. I study low back pain and lead a program that helps patients get the right treatment from the right healthcare professional at the right time.

Researchers and clinicians are still searching for answers to some of the questions that drove me to begin my career in science, but we know a lot more now than we did then. For example:

1. Low back pain, even when severe, is rarely caused by a serious underlying medical condition.
2. The treatment you receive for low back pain can depend more on the healthcare professional you see than your specific low back condition.
3. Most people with low back pain start seeing a medical physician first. However, prescription medications, injections, and surgery don't work well for most patients and can sometimes cause further harm.
4. Imaging, including X-rays and MRIs, does little to identify the true underlying causes of low back pain in most cases.
5. Nondrug approaches such as acupuncture, massage, yoga, exercise, and spinal manipulation work best for most people and are recommended by the American College of Physicians and the World Health Organization.

As I write this book, much of this information has yet to be widely adopted into medical practice. One reason is that new research results take time to become standard practice in clinical settings. Another reason is that many of the most effective treatments fall outside the scope of conventional medical practice. The result is that thirty-five years later, patients still struggle to find safe, effective treatment options or know how to access them.

I find this status quo frustrating and unacceptable. About three years ago, I decided it was time to go directly to patients with the information they needed to manage their own low back pain. I planned to identify a few great websites and one or two books. I would use them to create a brief reference list for patients with low back pain.

I began by searching the internet, and the scope of the problem became clear. I know it's not surprising to find unhelpful information online. Still, I was shocked at how bad the advice often was. Much of what I found was at best confusing, and at worst harmful.

Then I looked for books. I searched the internet and library databases. During my travels, I visited small local bookstores. Reading the books I found made me realize that many authors were not thinking holistically. There was no attention to diversity or differences in the origin of people's pain. Surgeons recommended surgery, physical therapists recommended physical therapy, chiropractors recommended chiropractic care, pain psychologists recommended cognitive behavioral therapy, and yoga instructors recommended yoga. Others shared the same narrow perspective I had found online, recommending treatments that the guidelines advise against. At least I now knew what I was looking for. A book that explains the complex causes of low back pain and how those causes affect patient care. A book that embraces the holistic Whole Health model of healthcare delivery, a model that starts by asking "what matters to you" rather than "what is the matter with you." A book that uses real-life stories and interviews with experts to illustrate essential points, that emphasizes self-management, and that makes low back pain treatment recommendations based on the best scientific evidence. A book that explains how readers can apply this information to their own, unique low back pain experience.

As far as I could tell, that book did not exist. I would need to write it.

Take Your Back Back is a field guide to empower you on your healing journey: part background information, part instruction manual, part review of the research, and part personal tales of resilience through pain. I've taken everything I have learned in the past thirty years, based on my experience and that of others, and distilled it down to the information you need to take control of your low back pain and live your best life. Part 1 provides the essential information you need to understand low back pain and approach it from a Whole Health perspective. Part 2 walks you through the many treatment approaches for low back pain. Here, you will learn which treatments are effective and how they might work for you. Part 3 is your call to action. It includes tips for choosing the right healthcare professional and a road map for developing a personalized Take Your Back Back Action Plan.

Your journey to healing low back pain is deeply personal. For you, healing may be a resolution of your pain or finding ways to live a full and productive life, even if some level of pain persists. There is no one-size-fits-all solution. This book will help you find your solution by empowering you to make informed decisions, challenge misconceptions, and embrace a holistic, Whole Health perspective. You will have the knowledge and confidence to pursue the treatment approaches best able to restore your quality of life. Whether you are new to low back pain or have struggled with it for years, real change is possible.

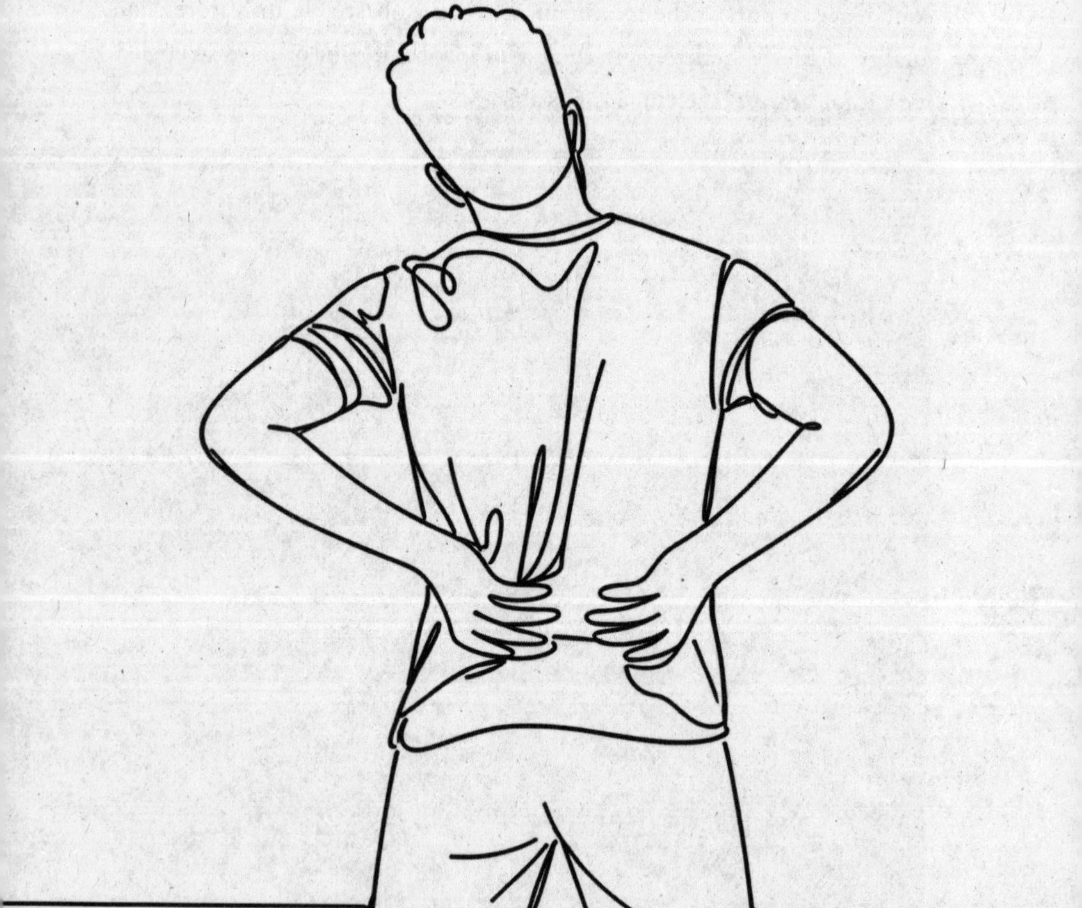

Part One

Low Back Pain Basics

chapter 1

Start Here

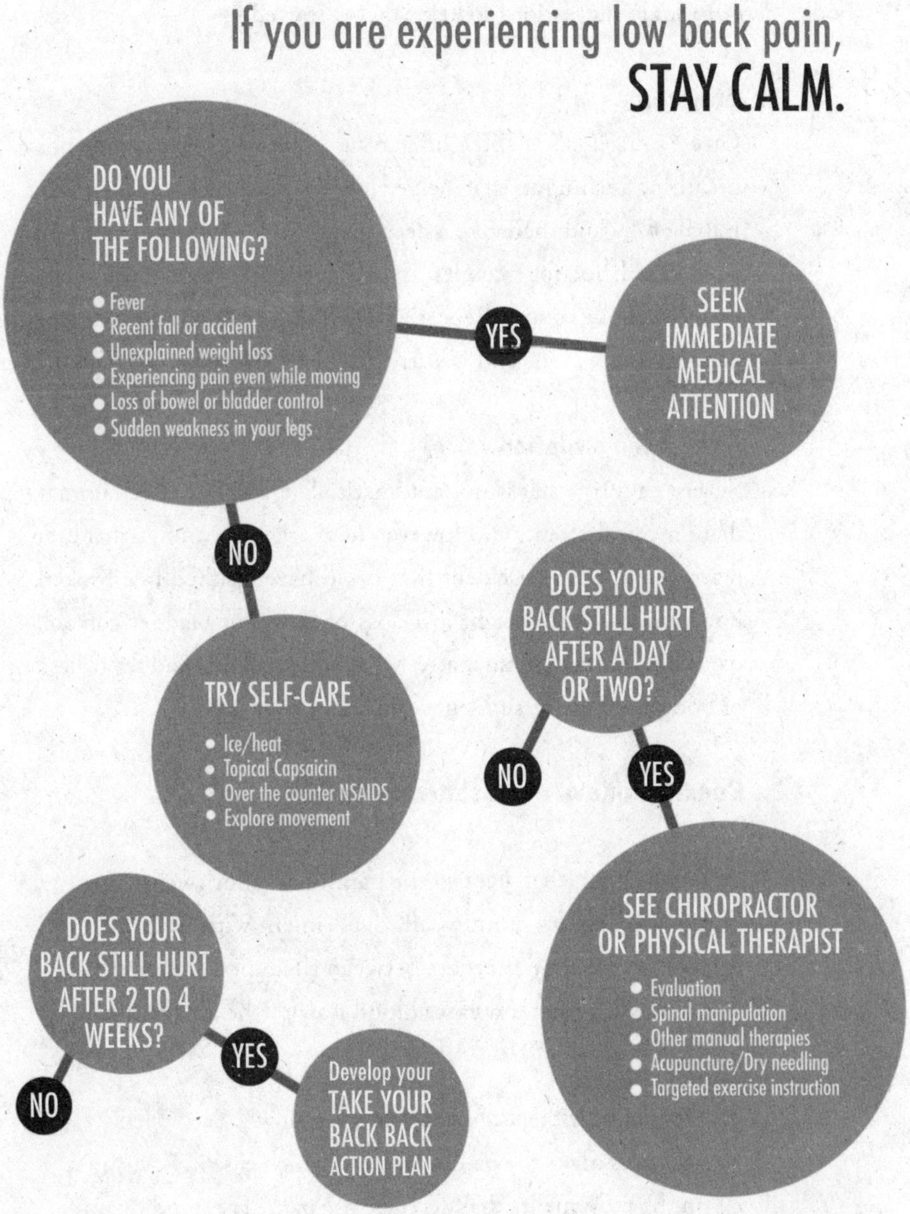
If you are experiencing low back pain,
STAY CALM.
DO YOU HAVE ANY OF THE FOLLOWING?
• Fever
• Recent fall or accident
• Unexplained weight loss
• Experiencing pain even while moving
• Loss of bowel or bladder control
• Sudden weakness in your legs
YES
SEEK IMMEDIATE MEDICAL ATTENTION
NO
TRY SELF-CARE
• Ice/heat
• Topical Capsaicin
• Over the counter NSAIDS
• Explore movement
DOES YOUR BACK STILL HURT AFTER A DAY OR TWO?
NO
YES
SEE CHIROPRACTOR OR PHYSICAL THERAPIST
• Evaluation
• Spinal manipulation
• Other manual therapies
• Acupuncture/Dry needling
• Targeted exercise instruction
DOES YOUR BACK STILL HURT AFTER 2 TO 4 WEEKS?
NO
YES
Develop your TAKE YOUR BACK BACK ACTION PLAN

Figure 1

If you are experiencing low back pain, it's time to take action. The right action, right now. You need to be able to function and read the rest of this book. Here are some suggestions to help you get started.

1. **Stay calm.**

   Give yourself some breathing room. Literally! The same box breathing technique that helped me so long ago can help you. Exhale fully and then take a deep breath in for four counts. Hold your breath for four counts. Exhale for four counts. Hold your breath for four counts. Repeat. Call a friend or family member for help if you are alone and feel stressed or frightened.

2. **Assess the situation.**

   Severe pain by itself is not automatically a reason to seek immediate medical attention. However, here are some things that are: fever, recent fall or accident that could have resulted in a broken bone, unexplained weight loss, loss of bowel or bladder control, pain that is constant, no matter what you are doing and regardless of body position, or sudden weakness in your legs.

3. **Consider one or more self-care options:**

   - **Apply either ice or heat** to the painful area for twenty minutes on, twenty minutes off. Experiment with what helps you the most or alternate between them. Ice numbs the pain, while heat increases blood flow to the area and facilitates healing.

   - **Experiment with moving your body.** Go slowly. See which positions make the pain worse and which ease it. Focus first on the movements that decrease the pain. Try standing up straight or lying on the floor and pulling your knees to your chest. Walk around for a few minutes. Your back muscles may feel tight, especially at first, but they should loosen up over time as you move. Focus on finding which movements feel the best and keep doing those. Continue to experiment. It is likely that movements that were painful at first will become less so after you begin this process.

- **Consider over-the-counter nonsteroidal anti-inflammatory drugs (NSAIDs)**, such as Advil or Aleve. Take as directed by the manufacturer's instructions.

4. **Get help.**

If the pain interferes with your ability to function after a few days of self-care, consider making an appointment with a healthcare professional who can evaluate your condition and offer guideline-recommended treatments for low back pain. The right clinician, often a chiropractor or a physical therapist, can make sure you are not missing something important contributing to your low back pain, offer additional advice about self-care strategies, and provide treatments you cannot do on your own, like spinal manipulation, acupuncture/dry needling, and targeted exercise instruction.

5. **Don't become discouraged.**

Expect your pain journey to be up and down at first. It can take several weeks for your low back to heal, and some days may be better than others. Stay focused on what is happening *now* instead of what you fear might happen in the future. Remind yourself that most low back pain improves on its own. Read this book. Develop your Take Your Back Back Action Plan if needed. Remember that you are not alone. You can do this.

chapter 2

Different Treatments Have Different Outcomes: Facts Versus Truth

Imagine standing in front of a large cupboard filled with objects that represent things others have told you about low back pain, and things you have said to yourself. To figure out what's in *your* cupboard, review the lists below. Check the boxes next to the statements someone else has told you about low back pain. These sources may include medical physicians, family members, friends, neighbors, book authors, TV hosts, journalists, and the internet.

What have you heard about low back pain from others, including your medical physician?

- ☐ Low back pain is usually caused by arthritis.
- ☐ Low back pain is usually caused by weak muscles or bad posture.
- ☐ A pinched nerve usually causes low back pain.
- ☐ A slipped disc usually causes low back pain.
- ☐ Bed rest helps with low back pain.
- ☐ Low back pain is unavoidable if one or both of your parents had it.
- ☐ An X-ray or MRI is needed to "see" what is causing low back pain.
- ☐ Corticosteroid injections cure low back pain.
- ☐ Surgery is the best option for severe low back pain.
- ☐ A medical physician is the best clinician to "fix" your back.
- ☐ Severe low back pain means go to the emergency department.
- ☐ Opioids are the most effective medications available for low back pain.
- ☐ Other: ______________________________
- ☐ Other: ______________________________

Next, check off the things the things you have told yourself or that you fear might be true.

What do you tell yourself about your low back pain?

- ☐ **I will be disabled forever.**
- ☐ **The pain will never go away.**
- ☐ **I must have a serious disease, like cancer.**
- ☐ **I will need to quit my job because of the pain.**
- ☐ **I will never be able to enjoy time with friends.**
- ☐ **I will not be able to take care of my family.**
- ☐ **Other:** ____________________ ____________________
- ☐ **Other:** ____________________ ____________________

Once you've finished this exercise, picture each statement you checked above as a label on an object sitting in your cabinet. Imagine each statement as literally and vividly as possible. Now imagine yourself clearing everything out of the cupboard. Use one arm to sweep all the contents into a trash can or carefully place each item in a trash bin—whatever works best for you. Carry the bin filled with everything you believe about low back pain out of the room, out of the house, out of your life. Now stand in front of your empty cupboard. Start putting new objects in it, each labeled with a truth. Here are some of the labels you'll want to include.

First, the general truths:

- Almost **every person on this planet has low back pain** at some point.
- **Most low back pain goes away on its own** in a few days or weeks.
- **Walking** is one of the best treatments for low back pain.
- There are **many things you can do at home** to treat your low back pain effectively.

- It is best to **try non-drug treatments** before prescription medication.
- Most people with low back pain **do not need X-rays or an MRI.**
- Experts **recommend against injections and surgery** for most people.

Next, add the treatment approaches that are currently backed by research and recommended by experts:

- **Spinal manipulation**
- **Acupuncture**
- **Massage**
- **Exercise**
- **Yoga**
- **Cognitive behavioral therapy** (especially for chronic low back pain)
- **Combined nondrug treatment approaches** (especially for chronic low back pain)

When it comes to low back pain, there is a big disconnect between popular beliefs and the little-known truths. Why does this matter? What you are told influences what you believe, and what you believe influences your actions. What you do can make a big difference in how much low back pain you experience and how long it lasts.

To see how these myths impact care choices, suppose your insurance plan believes the myth that corticosteroid injections work for low back pain, but chiropractic and physical therapy are not effective. As a result, they cover the total cost for a corticosteroid injection, but visiting a chiropractor or a physical therapist will require a $50 co-pay per visit. Some people might be more inclined to go with the injection because they assume the insurance plan knows best or because they can't afford the cost of a physical therapist. But as you will learn, experts advise against corticosteroids in favor of the treatments offered by chiropractors and physical therapists.

Or suppose your medical physician hasn't kept up with the latest research and still believes the myth that skeletal muscle relaxants (e.g., Soma or

Flexeril), benzodiazepines (e.g., Valium or Xanax), or opioids (e.g., Vicodin, fentanyl, or OxyContin) are the best approach for low back pain. In that case, you are likely to end up on one or more of these medications, even though the American College of Physicians recommends nondrug options as the first line of treatment. The truth is that drugs don't address the causes of low back pain and, as a result, don't work very well for most people. They can also lead to serious side effects such as internal bleeding, feeling sleepy, falls, and addiction.

It is time to explore some of the myths and truths about low back pain in a little bit more detail.

Myth 1: Low back pain is caused by degenerative disc disease, so your pain and disability will continue to get worse as you age.

The truth: On hearing this, your first response might be to feel frightened and discouraged, to restrict your activities, perhaps without even realizing it. The fact is that almost everyone experiences disc changes with aging, and movement makes low back pain better, not worse.

Myth 2: Medications are usually the best answer for low back pain.

The truth: Most medications used for low back pain are likely to cause more harm than help because they do not address the underlying causes of your pain and can result in significant side effects. As a result, both the American College of Physicians and the World Health Organization recommend the use of nondrug therapies, such as spinal manipulation, acupuncture, massage, and cognitive behavioral therapy, either before trying or instead of prescription medications.

Myth 3: Opioids are needed for severe low back pain.

The truth: Studies show that for most people opioids are no better than other medications for chronic low back pain and don't work any better than a placebo for acute low back pain. Many people who are prescribed opioids, even for a few days, are still taking them a year later.

Myth 4: An X-ray or MRI is needed to "see" what is causing low back pain.

The truth: Scientific studies have shown that people with osteoarthritis or a bulging disc often have no low back pain, and many people with low back pain do not have osteoarthritis or a bulging disc. As a result, in the absence of red flags, imaging is not recommended for low back pain lasting less than four to six weeks.

Myth 5: The emergency department is where I will find the best immediate treatment options for low back pain.

The truth: Unless you are experiencing the symptoms mentioned in chapter 1 and discussed in more detail in chapter 4, the emergency department is generally not the best place to seek care for your low back pain first. You could spend a very long time in the waiting room and end up receiving medications that the guidelines do not recommend, or unneeded X-rays, MRIs, or unnecessary referrals to pain specialists.

Myth 6: Surgery or corticosteroid injections cure low back pain.

The truth: Research shows that surgery often does not result in significantly better outcomes than nonsurgical treatments. On average, corticosteroid injections do not make people feel any better than a placebo. As a result, most clinical practice guidelines do not recommend injections at all, and surgery is only recommended in limited cases.

Applying Truths in the Real World

I have two jobs at Duke University. The first job is to research different treatment approaches for low back pain. Over the past several years, my colleagues and I have received more than $20 million in funding from the National Institutes of Health and other organizations. Here are examples of three recent research projects. The first study examined the effects of mindfulness meditation and acupuncture on patients with low back pain undergoing spine surgery. The second study evaluated the optimal number of chiropractic visits for veterans with chronic low back pain. The third study examined the outcomes and costs of asking patients who call to make an appointment with a primary care physician to see a chiropractor or a physical therapist instead.

My second role is to assist Duke Health in implementing best practices for the management of low back pain. I do that through a program called Spine Health. The primary goal of Spine Health is to ensure that the right patient is getting the right low back pain care at the right time from the right clinician. Accomplishing this goal is not as easy as it might seem.

Sometimes that right care doesn't involve a clinician at all. As you already learned in chapter 1, the best place to start for most people is with the things you can do on your own to prevent and treat low back pain. When this level of self-care is not enough, your options range from taking a yoga class to seeing a world-renowned spine surgeon. To help patients determine where to start their low back pain journey at Duke Health, we did our homework. First, we surveyed physicians and other healthcare professionals in our Spine Division to gather their opinions on best practices for low back pain. We then reviewed the research and current guidelines for low back pain. Next, we used this information to work with clinicians across various medical specialties to develop a care pathway for low back pain.

At Duke Health, many healthcare professionals collaborate to deliver high-quality, guideline-concordant care to patients with low back pain. This team approach is by design. Dr. Benjamin Alman, chairman of the Department of Orthopaedic Surgery at Duke University School of Medicine, explains, "With more than 11 million people in North Carolina, health systems need to provide easy access to back pain care that is as safe and effective as possible." He adds, "We do this by integrating neurosurgeons, physical medicine and rehabilitation physicians, physical therapists, chiropractors, and others into a single unit." Having clinicians with this broad range of expertise allows patients to know that they are "coming to a place where they can get the right care, from the right healthcare professional, right away, be that exercise advice or complex spine surgery."

For most people, the most effective and efficient place to start is not with the latest and greatest surgical procedure; it is with doctors of chiropractic, who treat patients based on known best practices, and physical therapists, who specialize in treating low back pain. Starting with chiropractic or physical therapy makes sense for several reasons:

1. These healthcare professionals are well trained to help you identify the factors contributing to your low back pain.
2. They can provide education and reassurance about the causes of your pain.
3. They can help you get to the right specialist when further medical evaluation or treatment is needed.
4. They can advise you on safe and effective self-care strategies.
5. They provide many of the treatment approaches recommended by low back pain guidelines, such as manual therapies and supervised exercise.
6. They may be able to help you recognize if you are experiencing depression or anxiety and talk with you about options for getting help.

Why a Doctor of Chiropractic or Physical Therapist Instead of the Emergency Department?

You already learned that unless you have red flag symptoms, the emergency department is generally not the best place to start when seeking care for your low back pain. Yet many people unnecessarily end up in the emergency department anyway. There are several reasons for this. Patients want to know the reason for their pain. They want a specific diagnosis for their symptoms. They want timely relief from the pain and its impact on their daily life. In many cases, patients have been told by others, perhaps by a friend, but often by their doctors or other healthcare professionals, to go to the emergency department if their low back pain lasts for longer than a few days. Dr. Rebecca Donohoe, associate medical director in the Department of Emergency Medicine at Duke University School of Medicine, has seen it all. Here she explains why many of her patients leave the emergency department with a referral to a chiropractor or physical therapist within the Duke Spine Health program.

> ***Dr. Donohoe explains:***
> *The most effective care for low back pain starts by taking the time to listen and understand each patient's presenting symptoms and unique journey. I need to ensure there are no specific symptoms or physical exam findings that require imaging or emergency care. The next step is to address their expectations and fears. Many patients arrive at the ED [emergency department] expecting immediate relief or a quick fix. Pain medication provided in the ED may temporarily offer some relief, but it does not address their underlying condition. Sometimes the medications can cause side effects, interact with other medications, or even cause long-term problems. I have found that if I explain how low back*

pain often can take a few weeks to get better and educate and encourage patients on conservative care, they leave feeling supported and less anxious. What really helps patients is knowing what to do next. Programs like Spine Health provide the care and structure that patients need and connect them to the right resources. We refer so many patients to Spine Health because it gives them a sense of direction and access to the conservative care recommended by guidelines. We have found that approach is so much more helpful than providing treatments that don't work very well or telling patients just to go home and give it some time.

Key Takeaways

- Much of what you've been told about low back pain is outdated or simply untrue. These myths can shape your beliefs and actions in ways that actually make the pain worse.
- Almost everyone experiences low back pain at some point in their lives.
- Effective self-care and non-drug therapies such as spinal manipulation, acupuncture, massage, and exercise—are the first-line treatments recommended by leading experts and organizations.
- Most cases resolve on their own.
- Medications, injections, and surgery are often overused, carry significant risks, and rarely address the root causes of low back pain.

chapter 3

Know Your Spine and Brain

The more you know about how your spine is put together and how your body processes pain, the better position you are in to optimize your recovery. This knowledge is especially helpful when you run into someone, perhaps even a healthcare professional, who starts rattling off phrases like *facet syndrome, degenerative joint disease*, or *bulging discs*. Instead of feeling fearful, you will be able to picture what they are talking about, ask good questions, and work closely with your clinician to make an informed decision on managing your low back pain.

As an example of how knowledge can help you make better decisions, meet my friend and colleague Stacie Salsbury, RN, PhD. Stacie was working in her garden and tripped over a piece of metal that had washed up during a heavy rain. She fell. The low back pain started immediately. The next day, she saw a chiropractor and described what had happened. He told her that she likely had underlying degenerative disc disease, and maybe the yard work was getting to be too much for her. When Stacie heard that, she told me, "I literally felt my world get smaller." Gardening is one of her passions.

While the details differ, I often hear stories like Stacie's from people with low back pain. A woman in a medical clinic elevator told me she could no longer walk up the stairs. "I just had an MRI," she told me, and then added, almost proudly, "The doctor said it was the worst spine he had ever seen." An acquaintance stopped picking up her grandchild because her medical physician told her she had degenerative joint disease, and she was afraid lifting twenty pounds would make it worse. A neighbor stopped mowing his yard after being told he had a bulging disc in his low back. These people made their worlds smaller out of fear. They believed without question what they were told about low back pain by clinicians, friends, or neighbors. If they had known what you will understand after reading this book, they might have felt less fear and made different choices.

Luckily, Stacie is a nurse who studies low back pain for a living. She understands how the brain processes pain from an acute low back injury and is familiar with her spine's anatomy. Her clinician's words did not frighten her. She knew she wasn't done with gardening.

"I said, 'Well, that's not really an option, right?'" she told me. "I'm here seeking treatment from you so that I can be in my life." She got the treatment she came for but rejected the potentially life-shrinking comment. Stacie used her knowledge about pain and spinal anatomy to stop herself from becoming fearful. Her injury healed. These days, she is still in her garden, doing what she loves best.

How Your Body Processes Pain

Something I hear frequently from low back pain patients is that other people think the pain is "all in their head." "All in your head" is both completely wrong and totally right. The suggestion that the pain is not real is completely wrong. The pain is very real. However, the totally right part is that all pain is processed in your brain, which just happens to be in your head.

Let's use some examples to talk about how pain works. You trip going down a step or spend an hour shoveling snow. As a result, you strain or sprain your low back muscles. Those muscles are full of nerve endings. Some of these nerve endings are called pain receptors. Their job is to respond to an injury by making your body aware of a potential problem. The pain receptors are connected to your nerves, which send the message to your spinal cord. The spinal cord sends the message to your brain. The brain takes over from there. It gives you an idea of where the pain is, how much it hurts, and what kind of pain you have. The brain also releases chemicals in your body that influence pain levels and trigger your emotional reaction and tolerance to pain. There are several types of pain. Here is a brief summary.

Types of Pain

- **Nociceptive Pain:**

  Nociceptive pain is a sharp or throbbing pain caused by damage to body tissues, including the skin, muscles, or bones. This pain is one of your body's protective mechanisms. Imagine accidentally touching a hot burner on the stove. Warning signals travel rapidly from your hand to your brain and back to your hand again. You instinctively jerk your hand away. Another example is pain resulting from a broken arm. You automatically limit your arm's motion and then seek help as quickly as possible to ensure the bone is immobilized and, if needed, set. You're most likely to experience nociceptive pain immediately following an injury to the muscles, ligaments, discs, or spine joints, such as after a car accident, a fall, or picking up a heavy box.

- **Neuropathic Pain:**

  Neuropathic pain is a stabbing or shooting pain caused by nerve or nervous system damage. It can happen due to the same type of injuries that cause nociceptive pain or gradual changes in the spine from aging or repetitive stress. One of the most common examples of neuropathic pain is sciatica, pain that runs down the back of one or both legs. Sciatica is often caused by irritation to the spinal nerves.

- **Central Sensitization:**

  A third kind of pain is called central sensitization. Central sensitization occurs when, for unknown reasons, your brain continues to operate as if you have an injury even after your injury has healed. In addition to pain, central sensitization is associated with problems such as sleeping difficulties, fatigue, and the feeling that the pain is too much to cope with. How much low back pain interferes with a person's ability to live their life is separate from the intensity of the pain. This is called pain interference, and it varies widely from person to person. Clinicians often ask patients to rate their pain on a 0–10 scale, with 10 being the worst pain imaginable. While some people have trouble functioning with a pain level of 3, other people can live a full life with a pain level of 6. Scientists are still trying to figure out why people respond so differently to pain. What they do know is that past experiences with pain and fearing the worst can make pain more challenging to manage.

Understanding Radiculopathy Versus Radicular Pain

Radiculopathy and radicular pain are two types of low back pain that have similar sounding names and some overlap in symptoms. However, as you will learn below, they are very different conditions that require very different treatment approaches.

Radiculopathy

Radiculopathy is a nerve or nerve root injury caused by disc herniation or severe osteoarthritis in the lower back. It is estimated that between 1 and 5 percent of people with low back pain have radiculopathy. In addition to pain, or even instead of pain, radiculopathy can cause some of the red flag symptoms you will learn more about in chapter 4—such as numbness and weakness in your legs. Seek immediate medical attention if you are experiencing these symptoms. Radiculopathy occasionally requires surgery to prevent permanent loss of lower-body function. In nonsurgical instances, it is one of the few low back conditions where some clinical guidelines recommend steroid injections.

Radicular Pain

Radicular pain, on the other hand, is caused by nerve root irritation rather than damage, and pain is the predominant symptom. Radicular pain is much more common than radiculopathy, and the treatment approaches differ. Instead of injections and/or surgery, recommended treatments include walking and exercise, acupuncture, massage, and spinal manipulation to help manage the pain while you wait for your body to heal.

Distinguishing between radiculopathy and radicular pain is difficult because both may cause pain and tingling in the buttocks and legs. If you are experiencing these symptoms, you will want to discuss the differences with your healthcare professional. When doing so, ask them to clearly explain why they think you have one condition versus the other. Sometimes, even clinicians confuse radiculopathy and radicular pain.

One of the things that makes pain so hard to diagnose is that there isn't a good way to measure it objectively. No blood test or device provides an exact pain rating. Someone can ask you how badly it hurts and how much pain impacts your life. But this experience can vary greatly from person to person.

Anatomy 101

So far, you've learned about different types of pain and how they impact your daily life. Now let's move on to some of the interesting stuff beneath the skin covering your low back.

The Bones of Your Spine

You have twenty-four bones called vertebra in your spine, plus two additional bones—the sacrum and coccyx (sometimes called the tailbone). The vertebrae start at the base of your spine and extend up to your skull. The vertebrae are divided into three sections (see figure 2):

- The cervical vertebrae
- The thoracic vertebrae
- The lumbar vertebrae

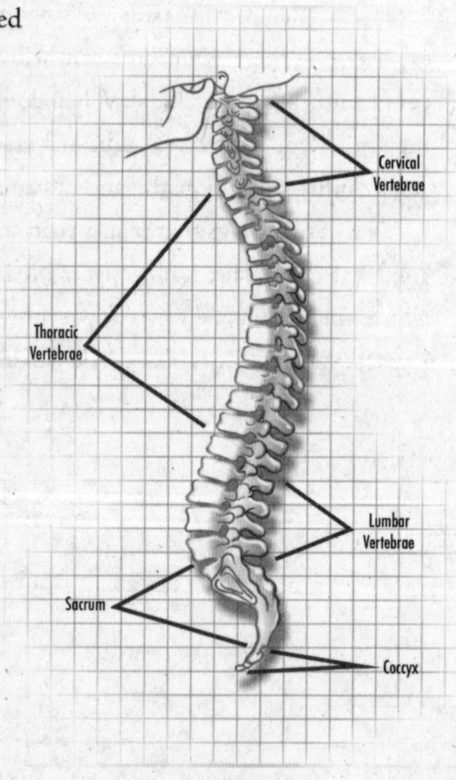

Figure 2

The low back includes the five lumbar vertebrae, plus the sacrum and the coccyx.

Vertebrae form a bony ring around your spinal cord and the cauda equina extending below the spinal cord to protect them and the small nerves that branch off your spine (see figure 3).

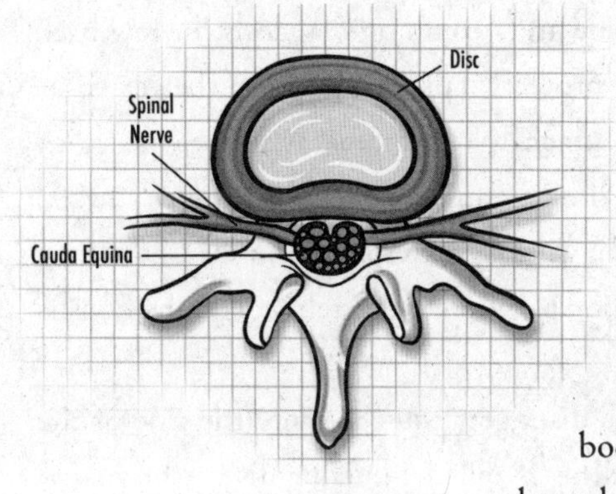

Figure 3

The oval-shaped front part of the vertebrae gives you the structure and stability required to stand up straight and move your body from one position to another. The back portion, known as facets, enables your body to twist and turn. The hard, bony knobs you feel when you run your hands down the middle of the back are called spinous processes. They help protect your spinal cord and the cauda equina, but their primary role is to serve as attachment sites for some of the muscles and ligaments of the back.

Joints called facets connect one vertebra to the next and stabilize your spine, especially when you bend forward or backward or to the side (see figure 4). As your body ages, your facet joints age, too. Sometimes healthcare professionals call this natural aging *osteoarthritis* or *degenerative joint disease*. Duke orthopaedic surgeon Dr. Joe Minchew once told me, "Low back pain is the only condition I know where normal aging is called a disease." The cartilage, a protective tissue between the facet joints, can become thin, increasing pressure on the joints. Osteoarthritis is both a common diagnosis for low back pain and a reason why physicians order X-rays. However, many people with osteoarthritis do not have low back pain, and many people with low back pain do not have osteoarthritis. While osteoarthritis can contribute to low back pain, it rarely offers the whole explanation.

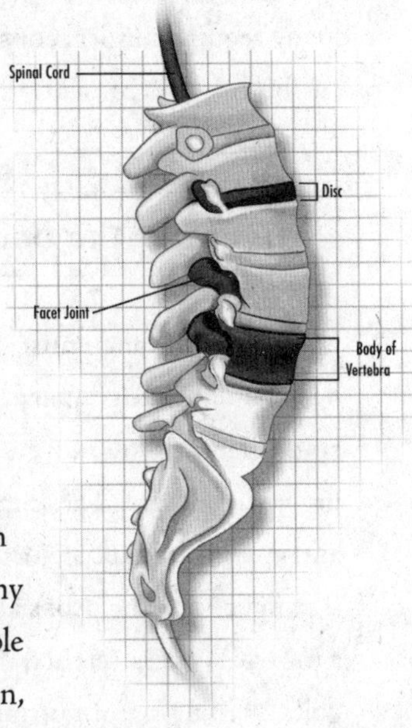

Figure 4

Issues with the discs of the spine are a common diagnosis for low back pain. Your intervertebral discs are protective pillows between the vertebrae (see figures 3 and 4). They help attach the vertebrae and serve as "shock absorbers," helping you withstand the pressure created when you run, walk, or stand upright. They're made of a gel-like material surrounded by strong fibrous tissue. The gel forms a cushion between the vertebrae, and the fibrous tissue helps keep the gel in place.

Sometimes the gel between the discs gets squished into the side of the fibrous tissue, causing it to bulge. This is called a bulging disc. A herniated disc—sometimes also called a slipped or ruptured disc—happens when physical strain causes tears in the fibrous tissue surrounding it, allowing the gel to leak. The strain can come from something big, like lifting the forty-pound combined weight of a car seat with a child inside while twisting to open the day care door. The strain can also come from something as small as bending over to tie your shoe. Bulging and even herniated discs will heal on their own in most cases. However, ruptured discs can cause radiculopathy and may require surgical consultation, especially if numbness or weakness in one or both legs is present.

Muscles of the Back

Muscle strain and muscle spasms are also common diagnoses for low back pain. Three primary muscles do most of the work in stabilizing your spine, helping you move your back in different directions, and maintaining your posture. These muscles include the multifidus, latissimus dorsi, and erector spinae (divided into the longissimus, iliocostalis, and spinalis) (see figure 5). The psoas also plays an important role. Strains occur when a muscle is overstretched due to overuse (common in some sports, such as golf) or injury (from lifting something too heavy). A spasm is when your muscles suddenly tighten. Spasms can result from overuse, injury (such as muscle strain), underuse due to excessive time spent on the couch, or emotional stress.

As the name implies, connective tissue attaches one part of your body to another. There are several types of connective tissue in the spine. Here I focus on three: ligaments, tendons, and fascia. Ligaments attach bone to bone, and tendons attach muscles to bone or other body parts. They hold the vertebrae together and connect them to your back muscles. A **strain** occurs when a muscle is overstretched. A **sprain** occurs when ligaments are overstretched or torn.

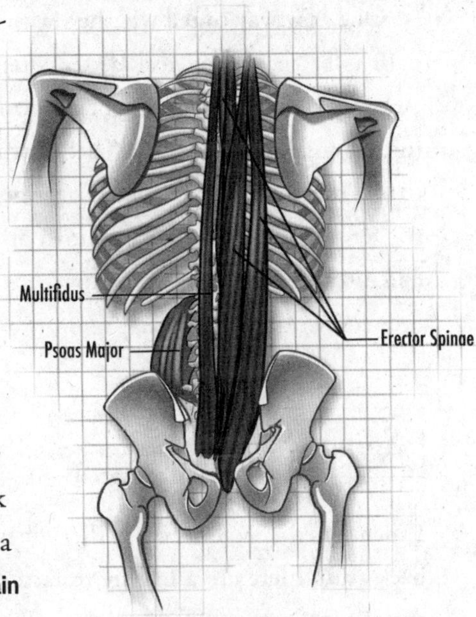

Figure 5

Your back muscles are latticed by a thin layer of connective tissue called the **thoracolumbar fascia** (see figure 6). Healthy fascia holds your body's parts together and helps them move smoothly against one another. However, fascia can become "sticky" and clump up, preventing that smooth movement. Sticky fascia can occur due to an injury, but the more likely cause is spending too much time sitting or not moving the body enough.

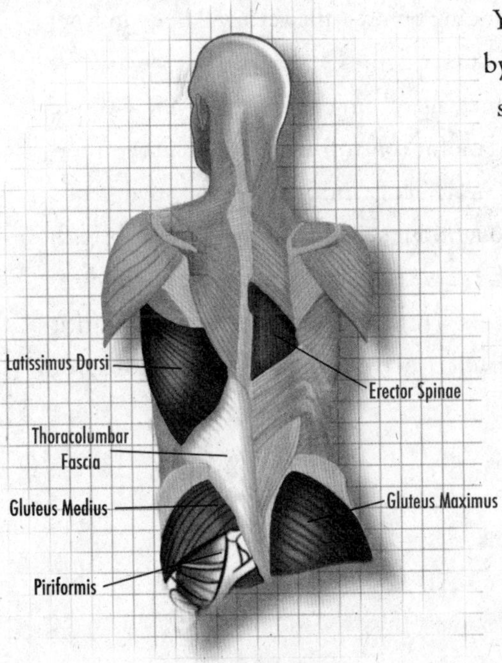

Figure 6

One easy way to tell whether fascia is playing a role in your low back pain is to see if you feel better after walking or stretching exercises. Another sign that fascia might be a culprit is if you have lumps or knots in the muscles of your back that hurt if you or someone else presses on them. These lumps are called trigger points. Your pain may be local to the trigger point area or radiate out to other parts of the body. Facet joints and discs are often blamed for low back pain. However, fascia may play an even more significant role.

Spinal Nerves

I mentioned spinal nerves earlier when describing various types of low back pain. Here are a few more facts that are important to know. The **spinal cord** is made of nerve tissue and stretches from the top of your lumbar spine to your brain. A collection of nerves called the cauda equina sits below the spinal cord. The spinal cord and cauda equina have several layers of protection: the surrounding bones—the vertebral body in front and the vertebral arch in the back (see figures 3 and 4). The primary role of the spinal cord is to receive messages from the brain that allow you to walk, jump, or bend over (called motor control) and return sensory information to your brain to register heat, cold, pain, or where you are in space.

These messages get sent through your **spinal nerve** roots, which branch off your spinal cord in pairs. The nerve roots travel near your facet joints as they leave your spinal cord. As a result, issues such as osteoarthritis and lumbar disc herniation can affect nerve roots if they cause pressure, inflammation, or damage.

Key Takeaways

- Understanding your spine's structure and how your brain processes pain can help you make more informed decisions about managing low back pain.
- Low back pain can manifest in many ways, such as a dull ache, a sharp stabbing pain, or a burning sensation. These differences depend on how your body processes pain and on what is causing it.
- Pain is processed in the brain. That does not mean it is "all in your head."
- The brain triggers your emotional response to pain and controls your pain tolerance.
- How much low back pain bothers someone varies widely from person to person and is distinct from the perceived intensity of the pain.

chapter 4

Diagnosing Low Back Pain

Determining the cause of low back pain can be complicated. Low back pain that lasts more than a few weeks rarely has a single cause. Instead, your pain's origin is likely to be a confluence of factors layered on top of one another. As a result, your low back pain journey is unique to you. It's time to explore these potential factors and why they matter to you and your healthcare team. The more you understand your low back pain, the more control you'll have over managing and preventing it.

Questions to Help Diagnose Your Pain

1. How Long Have You Had Pain?

Low back pain of less than six weeks' duration is referred to as **acute**. Acute low back pain, especially when it first happens, is usually caused by an injury to your muscles or the surrounding tissues. Repetitive work you are not used to, like raking leaves or shoveling snow, can lead to low back pain. So can a jolt to the body, like tripping over a step, even if you don't fall. Acute low back pain can hurt a lot at first, but usually after a few days or weeks, the injury will heal, and you'll be back to normal. While healing, self-care strategies (heat, gentle stretching exercises, NSAIDs) and guideline-recommended nondrug therapies (spinal manipulation, massage, acupuncture) can help decrease the pain.

In some cases, low back pain lasts for more than six weeks. This is called **subacute** low back pain. Pain lasting this long may indicate that factors other than the original injury are at play. It is important to identify those factors and take action accordingly. You will learn how to identify your "Back Factors" shortly.

Low back pain lasting more than three months is considered **chronic**. The causes of chronic low back pain are often difficult to understand fully. What researchers do know is that chronic low back pain almost always involves factors that go beyond the original injury. As a result, it may require more intensive or longer-term treatment.

2. Where Is Your Pain Located?

Low back pain can occur on either side of your low back or both sides simultaneously. It may stay in the same place or move around. It can also travel into the buttocks and down the back of one or both legs. In most cases, the treatment approaches for low back pain are similar regardless of where the pain is located. However, there are some important exceptions to this rule regarding pain that travels into your legs. I will go into this in more detail shortly.

3. What Does Your Pain Feel Like?

Everyone experiences low back pain differently. For some people, low back pain is an achy or uncomfortable feeling in the lower back that can extend up toward the mid-back or into the hips and legs. For others, low back pain is sharp and hurts so badly that it feels like any movement is impossible. Whether your pain is nociceptive (tissue injury), neuropathic (nerve injury), or a result of central sensitization (brain processing information as if you still have an injury even after the injury has healed) can affect how long the pain lasts and what your best treatment approach might be.

4. Do You Have Red Flags?

Although rare, some signs or symptoms of low back pain are associated with what medical professionals sometimes call a "sinister" problem. Let's review these symptoms, known as red flags. If you're experiencing red flag signs or symptoms, seek medical care as quickly as possible. But don't panic! Most people don't have a serious underlying medical disease even when red flag symptoms are present.

Symptoms / Red Flags:

1. **Fever and chills.**

   These symptoms may indicate an infection. Sometimes it's a coincidence that you get a cold or the flu at the same time as your low back pain. However, a fever may also indicate a kidney infection or an infection in the muscles or bones of the back.

2. **Unplanned weight loss.**

   If you're trying to lose weight, you could end up with low back pain because you have more energy, which leads to increased levels of activity—your basic "weekend warrior" situation. However, if you've had slowly worsening pain or are experiencing a new episode of low back pain and have lost weight without trying over the past six months, this could be a sign of something more serious. Keep in mind that stress and anxiety can also cause weight loss.

3. **Severe pain that never goes away.**

   Severe pain is a horrible thing to experience, but it's not a red flag by itself. However, if your pain is moderate to severe and never goes away, that is a red flag, especially if your pain is severe enough to keep you from sleeping at night.

If you're experiencing any of the following symptoms, go to the emergency department as soon as possible:

1. **Loss of bowel or bladder control.**

   Loss of bowel or bladder control can happen to anyone, especially as a person ages. I am not talking about a woman with three kids who has a little bladder leakage while doing jumping jacks, or a man who cannot reach the restroom quickly enough because his pain slows his walking. However, a loss of bowel or bladder control, especially when accompanied by numbness or loss of feeling in the groin region, may indicate cauda equina syndrome. This rare condition requires immediate surgery to prevent permanent nerve damage in your back.

2. **Sudden leg weakness.**
   In addition to loss of bowel or bladder control, cauda equina syndrome can also cause sudden leg weakness or numbness that makes it difficult or impossible to walk. I'm concerned about leg *weakness* here, not pain. If it's your pain that's making it difficult to walk, that's not a red flag symptom. Sudden leg weakness is a healthcare emergency even if you don't have severe low back pain.

3. **Moderate to severe pain following an accident or fall.**
   Like any other bone in your body, vertebrae can break due to a fall or other accident. This is most likely to happen if you have an underlying condition called osteoporosis, in which the bones are already weakened. Severe osteoporosis can even lead to stress fractures without a fall or accident.

Diagnosing Low Back Pain

Once you have ruled out red flags, diagnosing low back pain gets complicated. If you want an example of how complicated, type "low back pain" into any internet search engine. You will quickly find that different sources approach this condition in various ways. Some websites will tell you that low back pain is caused by low back strain, slipped discs, fractures, pinched nerves, arthritis, infections, or tumors. Others will discuss conditions such as muscle or ligament strain, bulging or ruptured discs, arthritis, osteoporosis, and ankylosing spondylitis. What many websites have in common is that they attribute low back pain to physical or structural causes. Low back strain is the same thing as muscle or ligament strain. Bulging or ruptured discs are the same as slipped discs. Clinicians and researchers aren't even in agreement about whether disc should be spelled *disc* or *disk*. And, while it is tempting for the sake of simplicity to equate low back pain with arthritis, osteoarthritis, and bulging discs, this is a mistake. Low back pain is usually more complex than these diagnoses imply. As mentioned previously, these underlying conditions are often found in people with low back pain, they are also (1) present in many people who don't have low back pain and (2) absent in many people who do.

If your low back pain is not solely caused by arthritis or a disc issue, what else is going on? There is no easy answer to this question. As a result, researchers and clinicians tend to use terms like *nonspecific, nonoperative, mechanical, idiopathic,* and *chronic primary low back pain.* Calling low back pain nonspecific or idiopathic means the cause is unknown. Nonoperative means a surgeon can't find anything to "fix." Mechanical means that one or more of your body parts, primarily the joints and muscles of your back, are not working correctly. Chronic primary low back pain means you have had low back pain for more than three months that is not caused by a serious underlying disease.

In early 2025, I wrote an opinion piece for MedPage, an online news source for healthcare professionals. The title of the article was "Five Things Patients with Low Back Pain Need from Their Doctors." I described what I had heard from members of the "Spine Squad," a group of patients who generously offered to share their lived experiences with low back pain with other researchers and me during a series of focus groups. A common frustration they expressed was lack of clarity about the causes of their pain. A quote I highlighted in the article was "They told me, 'It's just chronic pain.' That isn't a diagnosis. Something's causing it, and I want to know what it is." They also said, "Chronic pain is not a diagnosis. It's just a label they give when they don't want to dig deeper," and "Doctors don't always have all the answers, so we have to keep pushing, keep showing them data, keep refusing to just accept 'idiopathic' if that's not enough."

The frustration reflected in these comments is justified. Unfortunately, low back pain is usually viewed through the narrow lens of the biomedical model, rather than through more holistic models that may better explain such a complex condition. Below are descriptions of the biomedical model and an alternative approach, called the biopsychosocial model, which takes a broader perspective on health and healing.

The Biomedical Model

The biomedical model is the primary way in which the Western world approaches health and disease. The model is thought to have originated in 400 BCE with Hippocrates, the "father of modern medicine." It is based on the idea that health is the absence of biological disease.

I think of the biomedical model as separated into three components. First, all diseases are caused by germs or a breakdown in the physiological functioning of one or more body parts. These body parts are considered discrete entities, like a car with a flat tire or a burned-out transmission. The biomedical model overlooks the connection between the mind and the body, often also disregarding the impact of the environment on one's health. Many in the medical community approach the diagnosis of low back pain from this perspective. The problem with this approach is that it overlooks the complex anatomy and physiology of the low back, as well as its connections to the rest of the body, the mind, and the environment in which one lives.

The second component of the biomedical model is the patient's passive role. Diseases or disorders happen to people and require a medical "fix." This approach works amazingly well for accidents or acute illnesses, as well as for some chronic diseases. However, this narrow perspective does little to improve overall health or address complex conditions such as low back pain. Sometimes, following strictly the biomedical route can be a slippery slope away from a solution rather than toward one.

A third component of the biomedical model is reliance on "objective" diagnostic tests to verify the presence or absence of a specific disease condition. There are blood pressure cuffs to measure blood pressure and blood tests to diagnose diabetes. Imaging, primarily X-rays and MRIs, is the closest available objective test for diagnosing low back pain. X-rays show the bones of the spine, while MRIs and CT scans allow clinicians to view the bones and surrounding tissues. As a result, imaging can identify tumors and infections, as well as arthritis and narrowing of the gel-filled discs between the bones of the spine.

Imaging is widely used to diagnose low back pain. However, over the past several years, well-conducted research has shown that low back pain is often unrelated to arthritis or disc issues. Many people with arthritis or disc issues do not have pain, and many people with low back pain have normal images. As a result, unless there are red flags, most healthcare professional groups recommend against using X-rays and MRIs for acute low back pain. According to the American College of Radiology, "Uncomplicated acute low back pain and/or radiculopathy is a benign, self-limited condition that does not warrant any imaging studies."

In fact, early imaging is worse than not helpful. It can cause harm. Unnecessary X-rays expose you to unnecessary radiation, and both X-rays and MRIs can be a waste of time and money. Worse, research has shown that people who have early imaging have worse low back pain outcomes than people who do not. This may be because some people worry more about the causes of their low back pain if they see a picture showing "degeneration" in their spine. Another possible reason is that people who undergo imaging are more likely to receive unneeded corticosteroid injections and surgeries.

One of the comments I hear from medical physicians about the overuse of imaging is that they feel obligated to order it because their patients request it. This ask is understandable. Imaging allows you to "see your back" and demonstrate that the pain you are experiencing is "real." However, you are less likely to have pain in the long run if you avoid this temptation.

So, when is imaging a good idea? According to the American College of Radiologists, imaging should be considered if six weeks of guideline-recommended care is not effective or if red flag conditions are present.

The Biopsychosocial Model

In the 1970s, University of Rochester psychiatrist Dr. George Engel argued that the biomedical model was not broad enough to fully describe human health. He recommended incorporating psychology and social concepts into how one thinks about disease. He developed the biopsychosocial model, which considers how the combination of biomedical factors (age, gender, or arthritis), psychological factors (anxiety or depression), and social factors (socioeconomic status or job satisfaction) affects one's health. Other factors include the environment you live in, your ability to find accurate information to address your problems, and the emotional toll of living with chronic health conditions.

People who are depressed, anxious, or fearful are more likely to struggle with low back pain. They are less likely to respond positively to treatment, and their acute pain is more likely to become chronic. There are several reasons why this may happen. First, people who feel fearful or anxious may spend more time worrying about their low back pain. This intense focus may make the pain feel worse. Second, fear may drive some to visit the emergency department, see a surgeon, or request an MRI to "see" what's wrong. Research shows that these actions make chronic pain more likely. Third, fear can cause people to limit their physical activity, which is actually the exact opposite of what is needed. Finally, fear is associated with a factor that researchers and clinicians sometimes call pain catastrophizing. Dr. Francis Keefe, a professor in psychology and neuroscience at Duke University Medical Center and the director of the

Duke Pain Prevention and Treatment Research Program, talked with me about the role that pain catastrophizing can play in low back pain: "Ruminating about your pain, panicking about its potential causes, or feeling helpless in the face of pain are all associated with worse low back pain outcomes," he says. "If you are experiencing these feelings, there are a few things to keep in mind. First, don't get offended or beat yourself up if someone tells you you are catastrophizing. These thoughts are a natural response experienced at least to some degree by everybody living with significant pain."

Based on this discussion, I have stopped using the word *catastrophizing* because I don't think it is a good term to describe a natural response to pain. Instead, I have adopted the phrase *overly negative thoughts*, or ONTs. You will see references to ONTs throughout this book.

"Second," Dr. Keefe says, "accept that negative thoughts are a normal part of the pain process. Third, remind yourself that your fear itself is very real, but the worst-case scenarios you imagine have little or nothing to do with the reality of your situation. Fourth, the actions you take in response to these feelings are really important. Mindfulness meditation or cognitive behavioral therapy is going to get you a lot closer to healing your low back pain than a trip to the ED [emergency department] or to your local surgeon's office."

I have been focused on internal processes thus far, but your outer environment can also impact low back pain. The social determinants of health include your relationships with the people around you and whether you live with worry about money, racism, work stress, and whether you have a safe and stable place to live. These things affect your ability to navigate through life, which can have a direct impact on your low back pain.

Scientists are learning more every day about how dozens of biological, psychological, and social factors contribute to low back pain. However, it is already clear that a unique combination of multiple factors is at play for everyone. This means that the exact causes of my low back pain and your low back pain are as individual as you and me.

As an example, think about my low back pain story. I likely caused a physical injury to my back by foolishly trying to lift something far too heavy while twisting my body. That was the "bio" part of my experience. This would explain why my low back hurt for a few weeks but not for an entire year. Before my physical injury happened, I was feeling stressed as I struggled to meet the demands of raising a young child while navigating a challenging graduate school workload. I was anxious and probably a little depressed. That was the psychological, or "psycho," part of the model. I was experiencing ONTs that day in my biochemistry class when I couldn't stop thinking about how much my back hurt and feared that something horrible was going to happen. I was also worried about money and very unsure about my career choice. These worries reflected the "social" part of the model. All of these Back Factors influenced the persistence and impact of my chronic pain. Now it is time for you to identify your Back Factors.

Identifying Your Back Factors

I have described how the biomedical and biopsychosocial models influence our understanding of low back pain. It is time to sort through what this means for you. A distinct mix of experiences and circumstances led to your current state of low back pain. Knowing your specific mix of what I call Back Factors is critical to your journey. Some Back Factors are out of your control, for instance, factors such as height, past experiences with low back pain, age, arthritis, or disc degeneration. Once you acknowledge the things you cannot control, move on. Spending time on things you cannot change will only slow your progress. Other Back Factors are associated with your work. Any movement (or lack of movement) you engage in for long periods without frequent breaks can contribute to low back pain. This includes standing, sitting, driving, or walking. Other Back Factors are associated with your psychological well-being—stress, anxiety, or depression. Sometimes your Back Factors significantly impact how you perceive your life. At other times, they are barely noticeable. More on this later. Now, it is time to identify your Back Factors.

Exercise: Identifying Your Back Factors

The following tables list the most common factors associated with low back pain. Circle each of your Back Factors, underline the "maybes," and then indicate whether you think each factor has a small (S), medium (M), or large (L) impact on your life.

Back Factors That Cannot Be Changed	Life Impact		
☐ History of low back pain	S	M	L
☐ Arthritis in the spine	S	M	L
☐ Spinal stenosis	S	M	L
☐ Taller than five feet five	S	M	L
☐ Chronic diseases that cannot be cured	S	M	L
☐ History of a motor vehicle accident	S	M	L
☐ Vertebral endplate changes	S	M	L
☐ Radiculopathy	S	M	L
☐ History of disc bulge	S	M	L
☐ History of disc rupture	S	M	L
☐ Disc degeneration	S	M	L

Back Factors That Can Be Changed	Life Impact		
☐ Weak or tight back muscles	S	M	L
☐ High BMI	S	M	L
☐ Disc degeneration	S	M	L
☐ Smoking	S	M	L
☐ Depression	S	M	L

Back Factors That Can Be Changed	Life Impact		
☐ Anxiety	S	M	L
☐ Stressed/nervous/tense	S	M	L
☐ Catastrophizing (ONTs)	S	M	L
☐ Fear avoidance beliefs	S	M	L
☐ Feeling hopeless	S	M	L
☐ Unhappy with social life	S	M	L
☐ Low health literacy	S	M	L
☐ Less education	S	M	L
☐ A physically demanding job	S	M	L
☐ Prolonged exposure to vibration	S	M	L
☐ Sitting for more than two hours	S	M	L
☐ Standing for more than two hours	S	M	L
☐ Driving for more than two hours	S	M	L
☐ Monotonous work	S	M	L
☐ General lack of physical activity	S	M	L
☐ Not enjoying your work, school, or retirement	S	M	L
☐ Trouble sleeping	S	M	L
☐ Frequently feeling tired	S	M	L
☐ Chronic diseases that can be modified or cured	S	M	L
☐ Poor nutrition	S	M	L
☐ Nonsupportive environment	S	M	L
☐ Lower income	S	M	L
☐ Receiving workers' compensation	S	M	L

If you are wondering if your Back Factors include anxiety, depression, fear avoidance, or ONTs, ask yourself a few questions.

- Do you have trouble relaxing, often feel something bad will happen, or worry a lot? **If yes, circle "anxiety" in the list.**
- Have you lost interest in things you used to enjoy, or feel hopeless or tired all the time? **If so, circle "depression."**
- Are you afraid that work or physical activity caused your pain and/or will make your pain worse? **If yes, circle "fear avoidance."**
- Do you worry all the time about how much your back hurts, that it is going to keep getting worse, and there is nothing you can do to fix it? **If yes, circle "catastrophizing/ONTs."**

Note that this is a brief, basic screen to help determine what might be contributing to your lower back pain. It is not intended to diagnose or suggest treatments specifically for these conditions.

List all the Back Factors that you marked "M" or "L"—those that are having a big impact on your life.

Back Factor #1 ______________________

Back Factor #2 ______________________

Back Factor #3 ______________________

Back Factor #4 ______________________

Back Factor #5 ______________________

You will need this list when you develop your Take Your Back Back Action Plan in chapter 22. But first, turn to chapter 5 and learn why the Whole Health model may be the most effective way to tackle low back pain.

Key Takeaways

- Diagnosing low back pain is rarely straightforward because it often involves a complex mix of symptoms and events rather than a single cause.
- While acute low back pain usually resolves with self-care, pain lasting more than six weeks often involves additional factors that require deeper investigation and tailored action.
- Red flag symptoms—such as fever, unplanned weight loss, loss of bowel or bladder control, sudden leg weakness, or severe pain after trauma—require urgent medical attention, but most low back pain is not life-threatening.
- Embracing the biopsychosocial model helps us recognize that psychological and social factors—like anxiety, depression, stress, and life circumstances—play a major role in both the experience and the management of low back pain.
- It is essential to identify and address your unique mix of contributing Back Factors.

chapter 5

Introduction to Whole Health

In the previous chapter, I discussed the need to think differently about low back pain. One way to do that is by taking a Whole Health perspective. Whole Health focuses on overall well-being as part of a broader picture that includes physical health, emotions, daily life, and what matters most to us. This means more than how well your body parts and mind are working. The components of the biomedical model—arthritis, disc disease, muscle spasm—and the biopsychosocial model—fear, anxiety, and depression—are still important low back pain considerations. However, Whole Health places them in a broader context. The food you eat, your physical activity, the amount of stress in your life, how much sleep you get each night, where you were born, how you were raised, and the environment in which you live, work, and play also matter. The Whole Health model also focuses on who you are as an individual. By that I mean the things that matter most to you in life: what you value, how you spend your time, the thoughts you have, and the actions that you take in response to those thoughts. Whole Health asks the question, "What matters to you?" rather than "What is the matter with you?"

To illustrate how the Whole Health model can change your low back pain and your life, I want to introduce you to my thirty-two-year-old stepson, Jon. If you were to meet him, you might first notice Jon's slender, six-foot-three frame, quiet nature, and the charming smile he inherited from his father. You would never guess that behind that smile is a man who has struggled with low back pain, anxiety, and depression for more than half his life. The shocking thing? His family didn't know either. I have spent the last thirty years studying low back pain professionally. I know it affects almost everyone at some point, and I have firsthand knowledge of its devastating impact. I have written about the isolation people can experience as a result of low back pain. Despite all this experience, I still missed what was happening right in front of me until Jon came home for Thanksgiving last year. While he had casually mentioned having low back pain in the past, it was not something he talked about. He likely wouldn't have talked about it that day either, but he was in too much pain to hide it.

I watched Jon move restlessly about our living room, sitting on the sofa, shifting to a chair, standing behind the chair, and then returning to the sofa. When I asked him what was going on, he told me how much pain he was in and how similar episodes of discomfort had derailed his life for years, ever since a football injury in middle school.

In addition to the pain itself, Jon confided that the mental health toll from worrying about his pain was having a significant impact on his overall well-being. While the pain interfered with his life several times a year, worrying about his low back pain disrupted his life every day. Thoughts swirled around in his brain even when it didn't hurt. When would the pain come back? How bad would it be when it did? The result was periods of depression, anxiety, and stress, which in turn made his back pain worse. He was convinced that he had an underlying physical cause—maybe scoliosis or a structural problem with his hip—that his medical physicians had somehow missed. He worried that the pain would get worse over time until he could no longer do the things he enjoyed in life. He loved spending time with family and friends, walking his dog, following sports, lifting weights, and playing pickleball, but he was doing less of those things out of fear. He had seen a primary care physician recently for a complete physical exam. He hoped the physician would be able to find the cause of his low back pain and fix it. Instead, he was told he was "really healthy" and sent on his way. He did not know where to turn next. He had consulted healthcare professionals across various fields—including chiropractors, physical therapists, medical physicians, and a mental health counselor—but the treatments they offered provided only short-term relief or none at all. Even worse, he still lacked a clear answer about what was causing his low back pain and how to manage it.

A new plan of action was needed. I asked him if he was willing to let me help. He said yes. After years of frustration, Jon was committed to taking charge of his low back pain. He started by working with me to identify his Back Factors. They included fear avoidance, ONTs, depression, anxiety, stress, standing for long periods at work, trouble sleeping, weak back muscles, height above five feet five, and previous low back pain. He realized that many of his Back Factors were modifiable and noted the treatments most likely to help him—mindfulness, psychological therapy, exercise, and spinal manipulation. His priority was to decrease his pain in the short run. When you can't sit or stand for more than a few minutes at a time, you struggle to think about anything else. He chose to see a chiropractor as his first treatment strategy because he had used chiropractic successfully in the past. Plus, spinal manipulation was one of the treatments consistent with some of his Back Factors. The next time we talked, he reported that he "felt something shift" in his lower back when the chiropractor adjusted him, and the pain decreased almost instantly. However, instead of relief that the pain was gone, he worried about how long it would be until it returned. He was ready for a Whole Health approach.

Whole Health empowers you to live your life to the fullest by equipping you with the knowledge and skills you need to take charge of your overall health and well-being. This involves recognizing your aspirations and goals, understanding your current position on the path to achieving them, and then taking action to bridge the gap between your current state and your desired outcome.

Dr. Rowland Hazard, a Dartmouth physician and author of the book *Talking Back: How to Overcome Chronic Back Pain and Rebuild Your Life*, told me he has learned the importance of this approach through decades of research and patient care.

> ***Dr. Hazard explains:***
>
> *I'm convinced after listening to lots and lots of patients over the years that whether low back pain lasts for weeks or years, or how a person responds to specific treatments, has more to do with who the person is than what their MRI shows. The strongest predictor of patients' satisfaction with their low back pain outcomes is not their pain scores, or how much they could lift, or how fast they could run. It is the extent to which they were able to do the things that they told us pre-treatment that they cared about.*

> *Before treating anyone, I began to ask them, "How do you hope things turn out? Four months from now, what do you want to be doing with your life? What do you really care about? What would you really like to be doing?" Before a healthcare professional ever asks a patient about their chief complaint, they should try to understand who this person is and what matters most to them.*

The Origins of Whole Health

The Whole Health approach I describe in this book was initially developed and implemented by the Veterans Health Administration (VHA). Building on many of the concepts inherent in alternative health practices, the VHA launched its Whole Health Program in 2018 with eighteen sites nationwide. There were several reasons why the VHA decided to move in this direction. The number of veterans who battled chronic diseases, such as hypertension, diabetes, and musculoskeletal pain, was increasing. So were problems with obesity, depression, and anxiety. VHA leadership identified opportunities for improvement within their healthcare delivery system. They began developing educational information for veterans focused on self-empowerment and the need to take greater responsibility for health-related actions and outcomes. They made health and wellness coaching available. They also initiated peer support programs and expanded access to complementary and integrative treatments, such as acupuncture and mindfulness.

The Whole Health program is now used in VHA hospitals nationwide and is slowly being adopted by other health systems. In addition, government programs, such as the National Institutes of Health and the Centers for Medicare and Medicaid Services, are exploring how to incorporate the Whole Health concept into their research and payment models.

When I first explained the idea of Whole Health to Jon, he was skeptical. After seeking care from so many sources for so long, why was this the first time he had heard about it? That is a good question with a simple answer. Most health systems follow the biomedical model. As a result, these systems are either not familiar with or reject health practices developed outside mainstream medicine. Luckily, this narrow focus is changing as approaches like acupuncture, mindfulness, and manual therapies become more mainstream. For example, although acupuncture has been practiced in China as a core component of traditional Chinese medicine for centuries, it took until 1972 to gain a foothold in the United States. That year, the president's physician, General Walter R. Tkach, published "I Watched Acupuncture Work" in *Reader's Digest* following his visit to China with President Richard M. Nixon. The article sparked interest and marked the beginning of the acceptance of acupuncture, particularly for pain treatment.

Jon's next question was also a good one. He pointed out that he was not a veteran. "This may work for veterans," he said, "but how does that apply to me?" My answer was that the core domains included in the VHA's Whole Health model—eating healthy foods, getting better sleep, feeling more connected to the community, and seeing the right clinician at the right time—apply to everyone. Let's walk through it together.

The Veterans Health Administration Whole Health Program

As you can see in figure 7, the center of Whole Health is you. You are an individual, living in a state of mindful awareness, also called mindfulness, or living in the present moment. While mindfulness might sound difficult, it comes down to paying attention to two parts of your environment. The first part is your inner environment—what you think and how you feel physically and emotionally. The second part is your outer environment or surroundings. What's happening in the world around you can have a significant influence on your overall health and well-being.

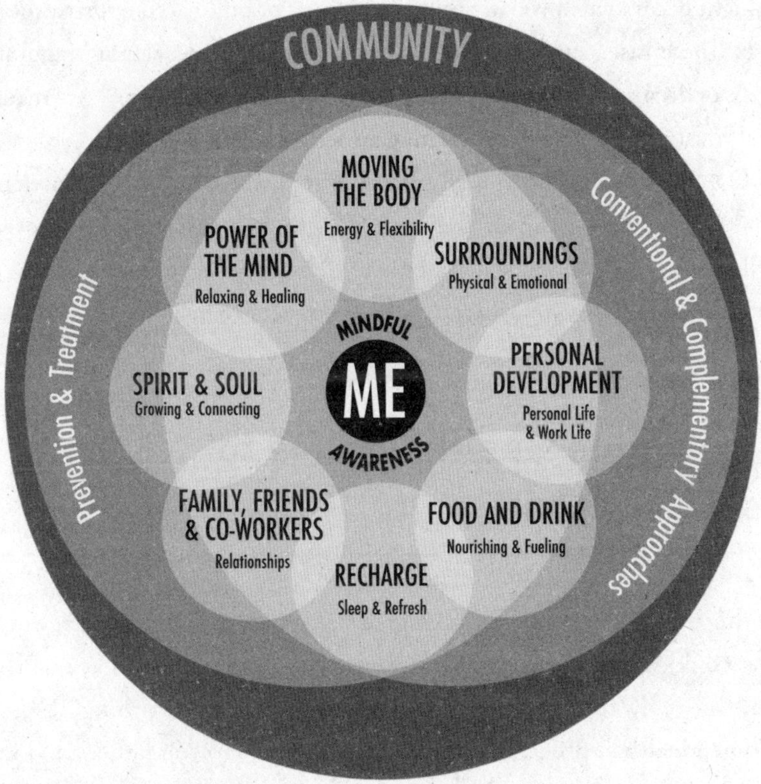

Figure 7.
Adapted with permission from the VHA.

Most people are familiar with the things that make up their outer environment—their home, the city they live in, and the people they socialize with. The inner environment is what goes on inside one's head. This is a world that no one else can see, encompassing not only memories but also thoughts, feelings, emotions, hopes, and dreams. This inner environment can be either subconscious or conscious. Subconsciousness refers to the things your body does without any effort. Some things can change if you pay attention to them, like breathing and your heartbeat. However, these things primarily operate in the background without your attention. The subconscious also includes all the information your brain processes in the background. This may include lessons from life events that you don't even remember, as well as subtle environmental signals like low-level noise, odors, or light. In contrast, conscious thought occurs when you actively engage your brain to accomplish a specific task. These tasks might include learning new skills, developing innovative ideas, or deciding how to spend your time. An example is choosing to manage your low back pain and then creating an action strategy.

One of the goals of Whole Health is to spend more time consciously thinking about ways to positively impact both your health and your overall well-being. This conscious awareness is an essential first step in taking the action needed to get you closer to where you want to be in life.

How Whole Health Applies to Low Back Pain

At this point, you may be thinking, "This is interesting, but what does it have to do with low back pain?" Jon wanted an answer to that question, too. My reply to him and to you is "pretty much everything." Using a Whole Health approach for low back pain can help you understand how your body, behavior, and mindset influence your daily pain experience and can remind you to recenter your life around what matters. As we talked, Jon realized how much time he spent focusing on his inner environment. He was fixated on his fearful thoughts, dwelling on dire future scenarios. This negative thinking led him to feelings of hopelessness and resulted in anxiety and depression, all leading to even more low back pain. It was time for Jon to become more aware of his inner environment in real time so that he could replace his negative thoughts with the positive conscious efforts required to manage his low back pain.

To get him started down the right path, I asked Jon to imagine that he was born wearing a backpack he would carry throughout his life. As time passed, his backpack gradually filled with the Back Factors he already knew were contributing to his low back pain. I asked him to think of his Back Factors as stones of varying size and weight, each adding to the total weight he was carrying.

At different points in your life, you will acquire or add new "stones." At other times, the stones will disappear or you will consciously remove them. The total weight of these stones impacts your ability to navigate through life. Imagine the difference between walking a mile straight up a hill carrying only a small light bag versus walking up the same hill carrying a backpack containing fifty pounds of stones. More than just the backpack's total weight matters. How much you can carry also depends on what is happening in your life. Your inner environment and surroundings—including your physical condition, the world around you, and the people you share your life with—also make a difference.

Think about walking that mile uphill again. Imagine how that walk might feel if you were alone in the dark, in the pouring rain, facing a forty-mile-an-hour wind. Now imagine that same walk with a friend on a warm, sunny day with a soft breeze. In both scenarios, your backpack is filled with stones. However, in the sunny scenario, it may bother you less because you are focused on the nice weather or an interesting conversation with your friend. In the driving wind and rain scenario, your heavy load may be all you think about as you climb the hill alone in the dark.

The bottom line is that during difficult periods in life, navigating your Back Factors may seem impossible. That effort may feel even harder if you are already struggling with your mental health, not eating right, or failing to get enough exercise. A vicious cycle can emerge—difficult life circumstances make low back pain harder to manage, and more low back pain leads to more difficult life circumstances. Jon realized that the biggest rocks in his backpack were associated with mental health—anxiety, depression, and ONTs. You will see in chapter 6 how this realization impacted his Whole Health approach to his low back pain.

The Whole Health perspective can help you short-circuit this vicious cycle. Maybe you are trying to figure out where to start. If so, you can do what Jon did—use the Whole Health model to learn how your pain can influence almost every aspect of your life. In that model, the first and most important question is "What matters most to you in life?" I asked Jon to start there.

Key Takeaways

- The Whole Health model emphasizes overall well-being, including physical health, emotions, daily life, and personal values.
- The Whole Health approach was developed and implemented by the VHA to address chronic diseases, chronic pain, obesity, depression, and anxiety among veterans, but similar programs are now being used elsewhere in the United States.
- Adopting a Whole Health approach for managing low back pain allows you to recognize how your physical condition, behaviors, and mindset impact your daily pain experience, encouraging you to refocus your life on what truly matters.
- Mindful awareness involves paying attention to the inner environment (thoughts, feelings, emotions) and the outer environment (surroundings) so that you can better understand the impact your thoughts and actions have on both your low back pain and your overall well-being.
- The rocks-in-your-backpack metaphor illustrates that mental health and environment can impact your ability to cope with low back pain throughout different phases of your life.

chapter 6

Whole Health and Low Back Pain

Overall health and well-being depend on the interaction between your mind, body, and environment. The Whole Health model breaks down these complex interactions into nine domains: moving the body; your surroundings; personal development; food and drink; recharging; friends, family, and coworkers; spirit and soul; the power of the mind; and prevention, treatment, and professional care. It is time to examine these domains in more detail, understand how Jon applied them to manage his low back pain, and begin planning how you can do the same.

Moving the Body

Movement plays a critical role in your overall well-being. This is especially true for those struggling with or susceptible to low back pain. Years ago, bed rest was a standard treatment recommendation for people with low back pain. Now scientists and many clinicians know that this advice is wrong. Instead, it is regular physical activity that helps maintain health and manage low back pain.

As Dr. Hazard explains, the most important key to handling acute or subacute low back pain is to keep moving. "This seems counterintuitive to most people," he says, "because we tend to think about low back pain from the perspective of the 'doctors can cure your low back pain biomedical model' rather than the 'keep moving so that you don't ruin your life model.'" Even a short daily walk can alleviate pain, improve mobility, and enhance mood. Because exercising is key to addressing low back pain, chapters 8–10 focus on incorporating this treatment approach more deeply into your life.

Jon realized that his job as an accountant, which required long days at his desk, meant he spent very little time walking or even just moving around. He committed to changing this but wasn't sure where to start. I recommended that he think about exactly what he hoped to achieve and introduced him to the concept of SMART goals.

SMART stands for:

- Specific
- Measurable
- Achievable
- Relevant
- Time-bound

Using a SMART framework to set goals and evaluate progress can help you stay focused on the actions needed to get to where you want to be in life. You will run into SMART goals again in chapter 7 and as you develop your Take Your Back Back Action Plan in chapter 22.

Two of Jon's first SMART goals focused on becoming more physically active—specifically, to be walking an average of ten thousand steps per day within six weeks and work out at the gym at least three times per week. He started small with his walking goal, setting the alarm on his phone to remind him to go for a short walk several times a day. He went a little bit farther each day when he took his dog for a walk. More movement helped his low back pain feel less stiff at the end of the day. Once Jon was regularly meeting his ten-thousand-step goal, he set his sights on the gym. Working out was something he really enjoyed but had stopped doing. He feared it would worsen his low back pain. He decided to work with a personal trainer one day a week and go it alone the other two days. The trainer helped Jon incorporate core stability exercises into his regular workout and gave him confidence that his workout routine would not harm his low back. The result was doing something he loved that helped decrease his pain.

Surroundings

The places where you spend your time play a large role in shaping your overall health and well-being. This includes your home, workplace, community, friend groups, culture, and values. Supportive relationships, calming environments, and a sense of belonging can help you feel stronger emotionally and reduce stress.

Jon loved his apartment, his downtown office, and his urban lifestyle. However, he did not love his part-time job at a local sporting goods store. Initially, he thought this second job would be a good opportunity. He could meet new people, enjoy the employee discount, and bring in some extra income. Instead, working evenings and weekends meant he missed being with his family and friends. Spending so much time with people he did not know was more tiring than invigorating. His low back pain was worse on the days he spent several hours standing in one place on a concrete floor. The income did not significantly impact his lifestyle. In the end, he decided to quit that job and focus on daily exercise, meditation, and time with friends and family.

Personal Development

Personal development is an effective tool for managing the stress, anxiety, and depression that can exacerbate low back pain. Perhaps most importantly, learning new skills or talents can also build your confidence and help you feel empowered to make other life changes. You will learn more about self-empowerment in chapter 7.

For Jon, personal development meant working to express himself more openly in his personal life and at work. His approach included several action steps. Talking to his dad and me about his low back pain and how it affected his life was a big first step. Reading the book *10% Happier*, by Dan Harris, provided new tools for becoming more aware of the negative messages he was telling himself and for focusing more on the positive aspects of his life. He used apps to guide him through meditation exercises. He worked harder to communicate his career goals and aspirations directly to his supervisors. This effort ultimately led to a promotion and a raise. Finally, Jon began working with a health coach, who helped him stay motivated. Jon found that the more energy he put into personal development, the less stressed he felt. To his surprise, he also experienced less low back pain.

Food and Drink

Hippocrates said, "Let food be thy medicine and medicine be thy food." More than 2,700 years later, science has proven the wisdom of these words. Diet can impact the body in both good and bad ways. Many chronic conditions have nutritional components, including cardiovascular disease, kidney disease, certain types of cancer, and diabetes. The traditional Western diet, which includes high levels of saturated fat, processed foods, and added sugar, can lead to an imbalance in gut bacteria. Eating foods that the body breaks down into certain glucose (sugar) by-products can cause systemic inflammation, leading to or exacerbating many health issues. In contrast, it is well established that diets focused on lean proteins, whole grains, healthy fats, and a variety of fruits and vegetables are much better for the body. Diets rich in antioxidants, found in many plants, can help protect against a range of diseases.

According to Carolyn E. Keeler, DO, MPH, physiatrist, physical medicine and rehabilitation physician, and assistant professor of neurosurgery at Duke University School of Medicine, low back pain may be on this list. "Systemic inflammation may contribute to low back pain by changing the way that the body processes pain," she says. "In addition, new research suggests that systemic inflammation may affect the intervertebral discs. While this is a topic that requires further investigation, I think about it when I am treating patients. It is possible that people on traditional Western diets respond very differently to injections than those who follow an anti-inflammatory diet."

While we wait for more data, evidence-based books on diet can serve as a good starting point for understanding the connection between diet and chronic disease. Examples include *The Science-Backed Anti-Inflammatory Diet for Beginners*, by Drs. Yasmine Elamir and William Grist, and *Super Gut* by Dr. William Davis.

I include smoking/tobacco use in the food and drink domain. Smoking is a Back Factor. Smoking less and quitting altogether both decrease the risk of low back pain. Studies suggest that smoking may contribute to low back pain because it reduces blood flow, alters brain function, and changes how your body uses and metabolizes vitamin D.

Jon doesn't smoke, and healthy eating was already one of his priorities. He didn't eat much sugar and enjoyed cooking healthy meals at home. However, after completing the Personal Health Inventory, he realized that when his back hurt, he was more likely to grab fast food high in fat content or drink a few beers in the evening. This pattern is a clear case of the vicious circle idea I mentioned earlier. As Jon explained to me, "If I am on a bad streak with my low back, I am less active. I also feel more stressed. Honestly, inactivity, stress, and poor eating habits go hand in hand. If I am in a good groove with healthy eating, I am more likely to exercise, and my back hurts less. If one thing gets out of sync, it is like the effect is compounded, and the entire plan falls apart."

Jon put this new insight to work, making a more concerted effort to stick with his healthy eating habits even when he was feeling stressed or his back hurt. Changing this habit was hard at first, but it became easier over time, especially as he began to see positive changes happening in his life.

Recharging

You are unlikely to get too far away from your phone charging cord, but how often do you think about recharging yourself? You need it just as much as your electronics do. Recharging is essential for maintaining overall well-being. This means taking the time your body needs to rest and relax. Quality sleep is critical to support overall physical and mental health. Poor sleep and fatigue are both important Back Factors. Adequate sleep and taking time to unwind help the body repair itself, reduce stress, and restore energy, all of which are critical for managing low back pain. When the body is well rested, muscles and tissues can heal more effectively, reducing inflammation and stiffness that contribute to pain.

Jon found that he slept better when he meditated regularly, kept up with his fitness routine, and put down his phone at least an hour before bed. He also realized that, as much as he loved spending time with family and friends, he needed downtime alone to recharge.

Family, Friends, Coworkers, and Community

Health is not just about treating physical illness. It also involves developing a supportive environment where you feel connected with others who are important to you. A sense of community can enhance your sense of belonging, reduce feelings of isolation, and help you stay motivated to make the changes needed in your life to relieve low back pain and optimize overall well-being.

In his bestselling book *The Blue Zones*, Dan Buettner found that a strong sense of community is one of the common factors connecting people who live long and healthy lives. A Harvard study that followed people for more than eighty-five years found that happy relationships are among the best predictors of a long, healthy life. Research also suggests that people who feel strongly connected to their communities have better outcomes for low back pain. Positive, nurturing relationships enhance mental health by helping individuals feel understood and less isolated. These relationships also reduce anxiety and depression, two important Back Factors.

Having a supportive network encourages individuals to stay engaged in their pain management plan, whether through motivation to exercise, reminders to take breaks, or simply offering comfort during difficult times.

Though this did not come naturally to him, Jon began to lean more on his social support system. This included sharing his struggles with low back pain and mental health, as well as his overall health goals, with family and close friends. Jon also joined a pickleball team, making new friends with others who shared similar fitness interests. As a result, he felt more motivated to maintain healthy habits.

Spirit and Soul

It is part of the human condition to want a sense of purpose, to seek inner peace, and to long for connection to something larger than oneself. To achieve this aspect of well-being, some people may turn to faith-based worship, others to mindfulness or meditation, while others enjoy connecting with nature or listening to beautiful music. These practices have the power to transform lives by providing a sense of calm and emotional stability. Jon chose to work on this domain by practicing mindful meditation each day. His practice helped him manage stress and foster a more positive outlook. He found that regular meditation reduced the intensity of low back pain flare-ups when they occurred. He also renewed his commitment to attend church every Sunday. Spirituality is important to him and something that he tended to neglect when his low back pain was at its worst.

Power of the Mind

If you have only one take-home message after reading this book, I hope it is how to recognize and harness the tremendous power of your mind. Research consistently shows that a person's attitude is vital in addressing pain and almost every other aspect of their lives. You will learn more about the power of the mind in chapters 7, 13, and 14.

To help Jon understand more about the power of the mind, I asked him to complete the VHA Personal Health Inventory you will find at the end of this chapter. The Personal Health Inventory is a tool the VHA created to help patients understand their current state and future goals as they related to the nine Whole Health domains. When Jon filled out the questionnaire, he was surprised to realize how much time and energy he had spent going down worst-case-scenario rabbit holes because of ONTs.

As I have already shared, Jon often worried that his low back pain would get progressively worse and eventually ruin his life. Becoming more conscious of these thoughts made a big difference. Jon started seeing a mental health counselor. After working with his counselor for several weeks, he found he could recognize these thoughts as they occurred and even steer them in a more positive direction. Jon's counselor talked with him about "rewiring his brain" to think more positive thoughts. For example, he told Jon, "If you feel a twinge in your back, don't tell yourself that something is wrong and start to panic. Instead, take it as a friendly signal from your back that it is time to get up and move, maybe to do a few stretches." This change was not easy, Jon told me. He had to stay vigilant to avoid slipping into old habits and thought patterns. But over time, this technique helped him address his ONTs and, by doing so, his low back pain as well.

Prevention, Treatment, and Professional Care

The Whole Health model approaches disease prevention and treatment by integrating conventional biomedical medicine with recommended treatment approaches such as acupuncture, spinal manipulation, yoga, massage, and mindfulness. While some of these treatments fall under the category of self-care, others require the help of an experienced healthcare professional. You do not need to be on this journey alone. See chapters 17–19 for information on choosing the right healthcare or trained professional based on your Back Factors. Sometimes that right professional may be a medical physician, a physical therapist, a pain psychologist, or a chiropractor. Sometimes it may be a health coach, a personal trainer, or a yoga instructor.

Jon's professional team includes a chiropractor, a mental health counselor, a personal trainer, and a health coach. Knowing where to turn helps him navigate painful flare-ups in the short run and build the skills he needs to self-manage his low back pain in the long run.

Complete the Personal Health Inventory

Now is the time for you to complete the same Personal Health Inventory that Jon did. You can fill it out right here, or there is a link to an online copy on the VHA Whole Health website. Think carefully about your answers to each question. You may not know how to answer some of these questions, and that's okay. Just complete what you can and go back to the ones you skipped later. One question that may take a little more time to consider is: What matters most to you? Think about this question carefully. You will return to it in chapter 7 when thinking more about the power of the mind.

Once you have completed the Personal Health Inventory, review your answers. Pay attention to the differences between how you rate yourself now and where you want to be for each Whole Health domain. Save your results. You will want to refer to them as you implement your Take Your Back Back Action Plan in chapter 22. I recommend that you complete the inventory again every three months. Do this without first looking at your previous responses. This will allow you to compare how you rate each Whole Health domain now with how you started. Also, think about whether there have been any changes in what matters most to you in life. The things that are important to you can evolve over time.

Healing from Low Back Pain Is a Journey

As you embark on your Whole Health healing journey for low back pain, it's important to remember that the road can contain both hills and valleys. The first two to three months after Jon adopted a Whole Health approach, he felt better than he had in a long time. He started thinking that maybe, once and for all, his low back pain was gone forever. Then, one morning, he woke up and his pain had returned. It was not nearly as bad as it had been at times in the past, but it was definitely there. He started worrying again. It would never go away. He was never going to be able to achieve the pain-free life that he wanted. The ONTs were back.

After a couple of days of overly negative thinking, stress eating, and isolating himself socially, he grasped what was happening and did a quick personal check-in. He realized that he had unconsciously skipped his meditation practice for the past two weeks because he was extra busy at work, had missed his last session with his health coach, and wasn't moving around the house or walking outside nearly as much. He hadn't worked out lately. He wasn't sticking to his healthy eating habits either. He began reframing his thoughts, reminding himself that he had managed to cope with worse pain episodes in the past and that this time he had the tools he needed to manage his pain. He started meditating again and worked with his personal trainer to temporarily modify his exercise routine so he could keep going to the gym in spite of the pain. He paid more attention to what he was eating and drinking.

Over the next few days, the pain gradually eased off. Now, after several up-and-down cycles, Jon knows the drill. He needs to stay focused on the things that keep his low back pain in check. When he feels a twinge, he slows down for a few minutes to think about how much movement he is getting, what he has been eating, and his stress level. Once he gets back on track with those things, the pain recedes.

What happened to Jon happens to pretty much everyone at one point or another during their low back pain healing journey. Dr. Keefe explains that low back pain flare-ups are common, and when they occur, it is normal to feel depressed or anxious or to experience ONTs in response. It is also common for people to stop doing the things that have been helping them effectively manage their low back pain. Dr. Keefe's advice when setbacks happen is to remind yourself that they have a time limit, usually lasting only a few days. Instead of getting discouraged or panicking, use this as an opportunity to develop strategies for navigating short-term flare-ups and emerging stronger. Those strategies may involve a recommitment to continue doing what you have been doing, but at half speed for a few days. Or it may be an opportunity to try something new.

Remember, low back pain is a very individualized experience. What worked for Jon in managing his flare-ups may not necessarily work for you. But there are things that will work for you—maybe you need to talk with your physical therapist about changing your exercise program or begin meditating for ten minutes before you go to bed. Flare-ups are a good opportunity for learning how to get back on track, a very important coping skill. Think of your response to a flare-up as a "behavioral experiment" from which you can learn even more about how to best manage your low back pain.

Whole Health is a whole new approach to your life, one that you need to sustain over time. It is not a two-week quick cure for low back pain. However, if you keep at it, the odds are good that you will have the kind of success Jon did. For more strategies on how to do that, keep reading.

Personal Health Inventory

Use this circle to help you think about your whole health.

- **Me at the center of the circle:** This represents what is important to you in your life, and may include your mission, aspirations, or purpose. Your care focuses on you as a unique person.

- **Mindful awareness** is about noticing what is happening when it happens.
- Your **everyday actions** make up the green circle. Your options and choices may be affected by many factors.
- The next ring is **professional care** (tests, medications, treatments, surgeries, and counseling). This section includes complementary approaches like acupuncture and yoga.
- The outer ring includes the **people, places, and resources** in your community. Your community has a powerful influence on your personal experience of health and well-being.

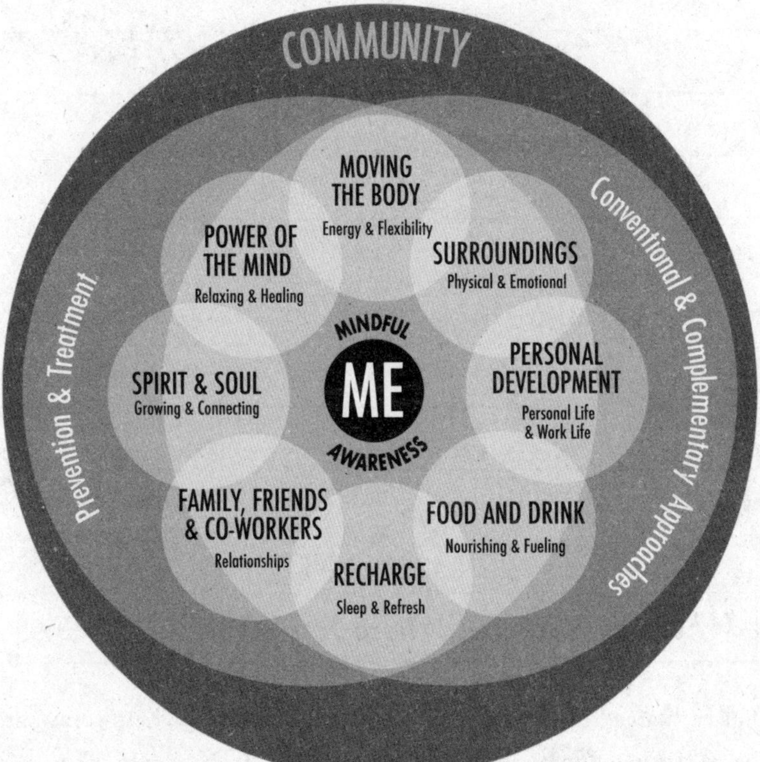

Adapted with permission from the VHA

Rate where you feel you are on the scales below from 1–5, with 1 being not so good, and 5 being great.

	Not so good				Great
Physical Well-Being	o1	o2	o3	o4	o5
Mental/Emotional Well-Being	o1	o2	o3	o4	o5
Life: How is it to live your day-to-day life?	o1	o2	o3	o4	o5

What matters most to you in your life right now?

Write a few words to capture your thoughts.

____

____

____

____

____

____

____

____

Where You Are and Where You Would Like to Be

For each area below, consider "Where you are" and "Where you want to be." Write in a number between 1 (low) and 5 (high) that best represents where you are and where you want to be. You do not need to be a "5" in any of the areas now, nor even wish to be a "5" in the future.

Building Blocks of Health and Well-being	Where I am Now (1-5)	Where I Want to Be (1-5)
Moving the Body: Our physical, mental, and emotional health are impacted by the amount and kind of movement we do.		
Recharge: Our bodies and minds need rest in order to optimize our health. Recharging also involves activities that replenish your mental and physical energy.		
Food and Drink: What we eat, and drink can have a huge effect on how we experience life, both physically and mentally.		
Personal Development: Our health is impacted by how we spend our time. We feel best when we can do things that really matter to us or bring us joy.		
Family, Friends, and Coworkers: Our relationships, including those with pets, have as significant an effect on our physical and emotional health as any other factor associated with well-being.		
Spirit and Soul: Connecting with something greater than ourselves may provide a sense of meaning and purpose, peace, or comfort. Spiritual connection can take many forms,		
Surroundings: Surroundings include where we live, work, learn, play, and worship—both indoors and out. Safe, stable, and comfortable surroundings have a positive effect on our health.		
Power of the Mind: Our thoughts are powerful and can affect our physical, mental, and emotional health. Changing our mindset can aid in healing and coping.		
Professional Care: Partnering with your health care team to address your health concerns, understand care options, and define actions you may take to promote your health and goals.		

Reflection

Now that you have thought about what matters to you in all of these areas, what would your life look like if you had the health you want? What kind of activities would you be doing? Or how might you feel different? What area might you focus on?

What might get in the way? How might you start?

Key Takeaways

- The nine domains of the Whole Health Model include movement; surroundings; personal development; food and drink; recharging; friends, family, and coworkers; spirit and soul; the power of the mind; and prevention, treatment, and professional care.
- Movement and regular physical activity are essential for maintaining health and managing low back pain. Even a short daily walk can alleviate pain, improve mobility, and enhance mood.
- Jon shows us how learning new skills or talents can build confidence and empower us to make other life changes.
- The Personal Health Inventory is an essential tool because it helps you better understand your overall well-being and identify areas that need more attention.
- The road to managing chronic, long-term low back pain is not always straightforward. It can be an up-and-down journey. During those down times, it is important to stay focused on your Whole Health lifestyle changes.

chapter 7

Self-Management

Self-management is a take-charge attitude that can help you achieve your Whole Health goals and successfully navigate your low back pain healing journey. It involves paying attention to your environment, being aware of your feelings, becoming conscious of your thoughts, and taking the actions needed to achieve what you want in life. Self-management matters, whether you're dealing with long-standing low back pain or experiencing it for the first time. The experts who create low back pain clinical guidelines are not always in agreement on specific treatment recommendations. However, they do agree that self-management is key in recovering from an acute low back pain episode and reducing low back pain over a lifetime.

Depending on where you are at with your specific low back pain situation, self-management might involve changes in how you think, feel, and act. These changes often take time and effort. Here are three mental tools that can help:

- **Self-empowerment:**
  The attitude or belief that you can make change happen

- **Resilience:**
  The ability to spring back from adversity; in other words, to keep moving toward your goals, even when the going gets tough

- **Sustained motivation:**
  Staying committed and disciplined over the long term as you work toward achieving your goals

Here I will describe each tool and explain how you can use them to positively impact your low back pain.

Self-Empowerment

> ***Whether you think you can or you think you can't —you're right.***
>
> —Henry Ford

Self-empowerment is believing in your ability to control your choices and take life-changing action. Studies have shown that people with long-standing chronic pain can overcome that pain by harnessing the power of the mind. According to pain psychologist Robert Kerns, PhD, senior research scientist of psychiatry at the Yale School of Medicine, when a patient believes that a treatment approach will be effective, that approach is more likely to work for them, regardless of what it is.

1. Figure out what matters most to you in life.

To harness the power of your mind, begin by thinking about the things you care about. I touched on this idea briefly in chapter 5 when discussing Whole Health. You answered a question about your priorities on the Personal Health Inventory in chapter 6. Now it's time to delve deeper into this idea with an exercise that helps define your priorities.

Take a few minutes to jot down three important things in your life. If "living a life without low back pain" is your top priority, write it down, then ask yourself why. For instance, maybe you want to spend time with family or friends, pursue your favorite hobbies, or devote time and attention to a career you love. Once you come up with an answer, dig deeper by asking yourself several times why it is important. Experts in this area say it can take five "whys" to get to the core of an issue.

Here is an example of how this works:

What matters most to me is living a pain-free life.

1. **Why does living a pain-free life matter to me?**
   I feel better physically and mentally.

2. **Why do I want to feel better physically and mentally?**
   I need to get back to work.

3. **Why do I need to get back to work?**
   I need to support my family.

4. **Why do I need to support my family?**
   Family is the most important thing to me in life.

Now you try it.

What matters most to me: ______________________

Why 1: ______________________

Why 2: ______________________

Why 3: ______________________

Why 4: ______________________

Why 5: ______________________

What matters most to me: ______________________________

Why 1: ______________________________

Why 2: ______________________________

Why 3: ______________________________

Why 4: ______________________________

Why 5: ______________________________

What matters most to me: ______________________________

Why 1: ______________________________

Why 2: ______________________________

Why 3: ______________________________

Why 4: ______________________________

Why 5: ______________________________

2. Assess your low back pain situation by telling your pain's "origin story."

To change how low back pain impacts your life, it is important to understand how you got to where you are now. You have already identified the Back Factors that influence your pain, but other, more subtle aspects often play a role. Now is the time to tell your story. Please write it down or record it on your phone—you will return to it later as part of your self-management process.

1. Start your story with the basics.

Please include any details you consider important about your low back pain journey up until this point.

1. **Where were you and what were you doing when your low back pain first started?**

2. **How long ago was that?**

3. **How is your low back pain now compared to when it began—better, worse, or about the same?**

4. **How is it impacting your life?**

2. **Pay attention to your thoughts about your low back pain.**

    1. How often do you think about your low back pain?

    ____

    ____

    ____

    2. What are you telling yourself about it? For example, are you confident that this is something you can overcome, or are you convinced it will last forever? Do you think the pain will improve over time or worsen?

    ____

    ____

    ____

3. **Think about the myths and truths you learned about in chapter 2.**

    1. Which myths do you believe in?

    ____

    ____

    ____

    2. Which truths were new information?

    ____

    ____

    ____

3. How much stress/anxiety/depression are you experiencing? Was it present before your low back pain started, or is it new?

____

____

____

3. Identify the obstacles you face and your strengths to overcome them.

Once you have recognized what matters most to you and assessed your low back pain situation, it is time to identify (1) the obstacles you face in implementing any necessary changes and (2) the strengths you have to overcome those obstacles.

Obstacles

Many people who have had low back pain for a long time feel helpless. Others feel hopeless or fearful. Still others feel anxious, depressed, or stressed. You may be experiencing one or all of these emotions, which can feel like major obstacles at times.

Additional obstacles include personal habits such as overwork, poor diet, lack of physical activity, low social engagement, or smoking. Examples of logistical obstacles include the distance from your home to the office of the right healthcare professional, lack of transportation, lack of time, and financial resources.

Write down at least three obstacles you face.

Try to include at least one emotional obstacle, one personal habit getting in your way, and one logistical obstacle.

1. ______________________________

2. ______________________________

3. ______________________________

4. ______________________________

5. ______________________________

6. ______________________________

Strengths

Strength number one. You are the expert on your low back pain. No one knows your low back pain better than you do—how it feels, what treatment you have tried, what works, what doesn't, and how it impacts your life. You decide what to do first when the pain starts, from doing nothing to trying an ice pack to taking an Advil. You decide what healthcare professionals to see, when to see them, and whether you will follow their treatment recommendations.

Additional strengths can come from many corners. They may include the support of family and friends. You many find strength in how much you enjoy spending time at work, going to school, or in retirement. Your habits and attitude can also be strengths, including a good sleep schedule, a healthy diet, regular exercise, and a positive outlook on life.

Write down your strengths here.

You can begin with three that apply to almost everyone.

1. I understand how low back pain impacts my life better than anyone else.

2. My body is stronger and more capable than I think.

3. My mind is stronger and more capable than I realize.

4. ____

5. ____

6. ____

Next, compare your list of obstacles with your list of strengths.

Consider how you can leverage your strengths to overcome obstacles. Add your obstacles and strengths to your low back pain story. Remember, you are starting at wherever you are right now, and that's okay. The goal is to move forward from there. How fast or far is not as important as consistently going in the right direction. You will set yourself up to fail if you start with unrealistic expectations. Instead, think about climbing slowly up a ladder toward your goal, taking it one step at a time. You will focus more on goal setting when you develop your Take Your Back Back Action Plan in chapter 22.

____

____

____

____

____

____

____

____

Resilience

> ***It's your reaction to adversity, not adversity itself, that determines how your life's story will develop.***
>
> —Dieter F. Uchtdorf

Resilience is the ability to recover, or "bounce back," when bad things happen. While everyone has different levels of built-in resilience, it is a learned ability that can be developed with patience.

There are two ways that resilience impacts low back pain. How one interprets that initial shock of pain sets the stage for first actions, whether that is a rush to the emergency department or making an appointment with a physical therapist. Your first reaction can determine whether your low back pain lasts for days or years. Imagine you are lying on the floor writhing in pain. A response of "Wow, this sucks. Someone bring me an ice pack and some Advil so I can get up off the floor and visit the physical therapist," is different from reaching for your phone to call an ambulance. Resilience is especially critical when dealing with long-lasting chronic low back pain. It might not decrease pain levels per se, but it has a significant impact on how well people function despite their pain.

There are many ways to build resilience, and they mostly align with the lifestyle activities recommended by the Whole Health model. Higher levels of resilience are associated with recharging, focusing on personal development, eating healthy foods, and engaging in physical activity. It is also essential to set clear goals for yourself, work to achieve them, and maintain a positive attitude during the process.

Part of developing resilience involves learning to cultivate a positive attitude toward yourself. You may have heard people described as thinking of life from either the "glass half full or glass half empty" perspective. Which are you when it comes to your low back pain? Read your low back pain story again for clues in the messages or stories you are telling yourself. Are those stories mostly positive or mostly negative? If you are spending a lot of time on negative thoughts, consider how you can reframe those thoughts. There are several ways to do this.

As a first step, notice your thoughts as Jon did in chapter 6. You can't consciously work on changing something you are unaware of. Keeping a journal can help you pay more attention to your thoughts. Journaling itself is thought to increase resilience. You already began this process by writing your low back pain story. Consider adding more to your story each day, focusing on your personal experience with low back pain. Include your action steps, what you learned along the way, frustrations, and wins. Journaling helps you become more aware of your thoughts and helps you think differently about what is happening in your life. Writing things down can also help you remember details that may be important when you talk with healthcare professionals about your pain. Maintaining a written record of your progress over time reminds you of your growing resilience and helps to identify what worked (and what didn't) for your low back pain. Perhaps most importantly, journaling can also help you focus on gratitude. To learn more about the benefits and strategies of journaling, consider reading *The Artist's Way*, by Julia Cameron, and *The Book of Alchemy*, by Suleika Jaouad.

Scientists have linked gratitude with developing resilience and positive health outcomes. A recent study found that older adults with chronic low back pain who reported higher levels of gratitude were less likely to be stressed or depressed and had less trouble sleeping. When you are in pain, thinking about gratitude can be tough. Begin by thinking about three things you are grateful for right now. Focus on the big and small things. I do this every morning, right after I get out of bed. This morning, my three things included: a good night's sleep, seventy-degree days in March, and my job. Write about the things you are grateful for in your journal. If you are having trouble wrapping your head around how to incorporate gratitude into your life, consider checking out the free thirty-day gratitude program available online through the Mayo Clinic.

Sustained Motivation

> **Some people want it to happen, some wish it would happen, others make it happen.**
>
> —Michael Jordan

By now, you have learned that healing your low back pain may require effort. You may need to make long-lasting changes in your life. Some days this feels easy. Other days, this may seem almost impossible. This is where sustained motivation comes in. Motivation is the driving force behind taking the action required to achieve our goals in life. Sustained means you are in it for the long haul.

To help us better understand motivation, experts distinguish between intrinsic and extrinsic motivation. Intrinsic motivation is when you do something because it feels good. The feelings you experience while engaged in the behavior itself are the reward. For example, working at a job you enjoy because you feel like you make a difference or because you love interacting with your colleagues. Extrinsic motivation is when you engage in behavior to obtain an external reward. For example, working at a job because you need a paycheck. Both internal and external motivators can help you tackle your low back pain in the long run.

Here are a few examples of intrinsic and extrinsic motivation.

Intrinsic motivation:

- **Go for a walk** two times per week with your best friend because it is something you really look forward to doing.
- **Prepare healthy meals** because you love to cook.
- **Attend church services** regularly because doing so brings you a sense of peace.

Extrinsic motivation:

- **Set small, achievable, and incremental goals** based on your "why." You want to walk five thousand steps, not because you love walking, but because it will help decrease your low back pain.
- **Focus on one thing and then do it**, even when you don't feel like it. No excuses. Make an appointment with a chiropractor or physical therapist. Keep the appointment. Pick one self-care option. Incorporate it into your daily routine.
- **Meet your milestones** because you know you will have an excuse to celebrate with friends and family once you do so.

Do some self-exploration to learn more about intrinsic motivation and which tactics work best for staying motivated over long periods. If you want to learn more about motivation, there are several books you can consider picking up. These include *Atomic Habits,* by James Clear; *Scarcity Brain,* by Michael Easter; *The Power of Discipline,* by Daniel Walter; *Tiny Habits,* by B. J. Fogg; and *Do the Hard Things First,* by Scott Allan.

Healing low back pain requires sustained motivation through consistent effort over time. Sometimes you will need to do things you really don't feel like doing. Do them anyway. The reward is worth the effort. If you don't believe me, just ask Chris.

I sat next to Chris at a meeting sponsored by the Chronic Pain Centre of Excellence for Canadian Veterans, an organization supporting research on Canadian veterans with chronic pain. Every year, the Centre brings together researchers, clinicians, and veterans like Chris. One goal of this meeting is to learn from veterans as they describe their lived experiences with chronic pain. Chris, a veteran of the war in Bosnia, looks like a pretty tough guy. His tattooed upper arms are as big as tree trunks. You would never guess that he lives daily with chronic low back pain.

Here is Chris' story:

How I injured my lower back was not even in a cool way. I was deployed on a peacekeeping operation during the winter. One night, I slipped on an ice-covered step as I was leaving the mess hall. I skidded down three steps and landed on my feet, but hard on the ground. Whew, I told myself. That was close. I went back to the barracks and climbed into bed. The next morning, I woke up screaming in pain. My roommate had to carry me to the medical clinic. There the doctor told me, "Hey, your back's never going to recover more than 80 percent. Learn to live with that." It played with my head a bit, at first, but then I was like, no, I'm going to be better than that.

I wish I could go back and find that doc now. Because twenty-three years later, I can pull 405 pounds in a dead lift. However, there are days when I grab onto that bar, and it feels like somebody's nailed it to the ground. On days like that, I'm not going to force it. I tell myself maybe today's not the day that I deadlift. A lot of us got injured in military training because we were taught, "Suck it up, soldier." Even if you have a broken foot. That's not resilience. That's pushing yourself to the point of failure by going beyond your limitations.

Real resilience is being adaptive. Know your limitations and optimize the functionality you have. I learned that by figuring out where that limit is every day, and then making a plan from there, you're training yourself to push past it eventually. You can still live your life with chronic back pain.

What Chris reminded me is that action—provided it is the right action at the right time—is the foundation for addressing low back pain. As he told me, "Everybody is capable of something. I can't do X, but I can do Y. So I do Y. I might wake up and think, today's the day I am cleaning this whole house. And then [the pain] may be like, Hmm, joke's on you. You're not doing that. Okay. But I can do the laundry. I can reach over my head and dust. Maybe that job doesn't get done all at once. Some days it's incremental. And that's okay."

So far, I have focused on the basics of low back pain—understanding the difference between facts and myths, low back anatomy, how the body processes pain, the Whole Health model, and self-management fundamentals. I started there because these are the building blocks for managing your low back pain effectively. Now it is time to move on to Part 2, where I will cover an equally critical component of managing low back pain—choosing your treatment approach. Chapters 8–17 describe many of the treatments commonly used for low back pain. You will learn which treatments are most often recommended by experts, which are best only in specific situations, and which are not recommended at all.

It's time to get started.

Key Takeaways

- Self-management is fundamental to achieving success during the low back pain healing journey.
- Effective self-management involves changing how you think, feel, and act. This requires self-empowerment, resilience, and sustained motivation.
- Identifying your obstacles and strengths and understanding how they relate to one another will empower you to develop a plan to overcome the obstacles.
- Setting clear and achievable goals is essential. Focusing on three or fewer goals at a time can help you avoid feeling overwhelmed and set you up for success.
- Building resilience is crucial for dealing with long-lasting chronic low back pain. This can be achieved by maintaining a positive attitude and incorporating gratitude into your life.

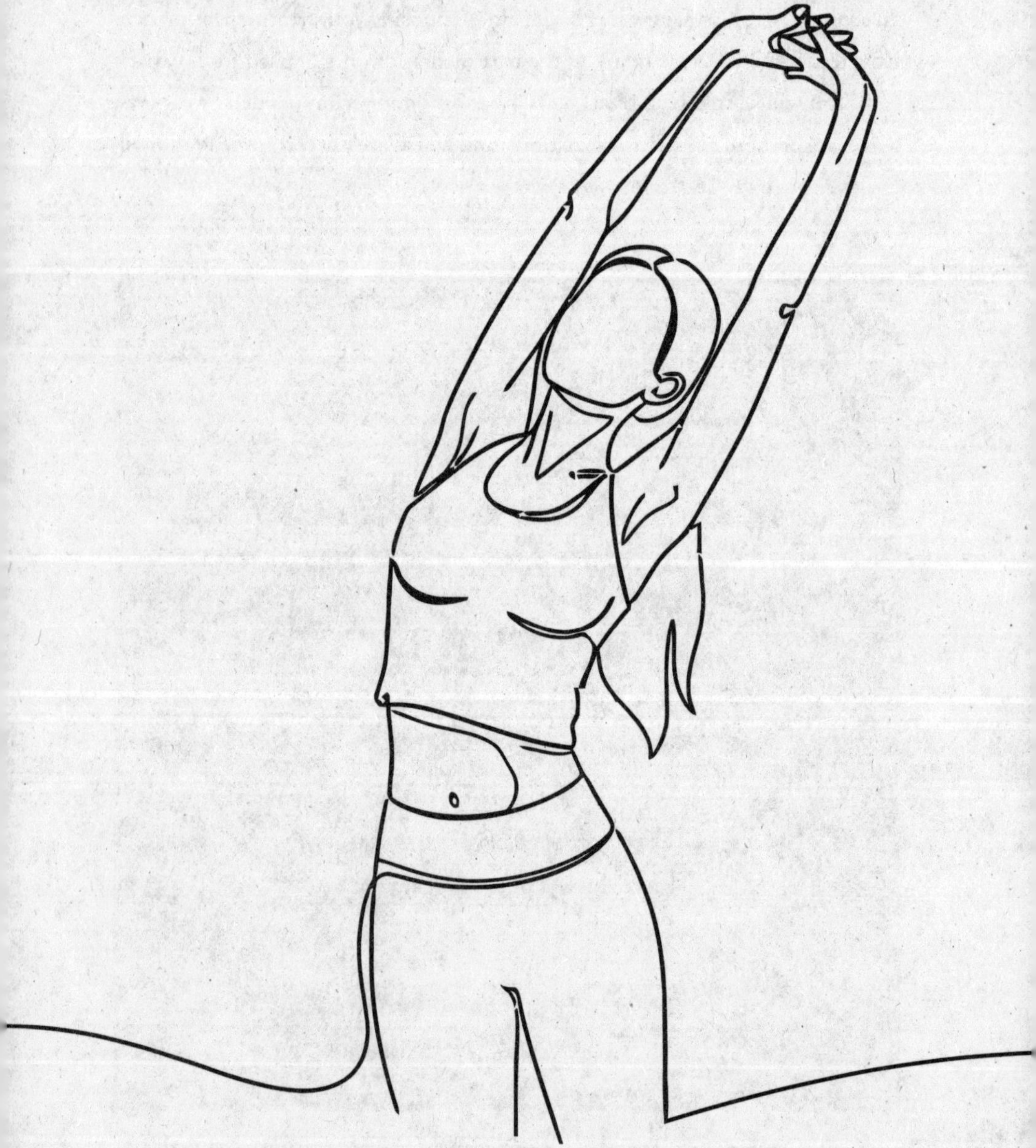

Part Two

Treatment Approaches for Low Back Pain

chapter 8

An Introduction to Exercise

If you are seeking a miracle cure for low back pain, you are not alone. Trying to find that one thing that will finally make the pain go away drives many toward imaging, injections, prescription medications, and surgical procedures. Unfortunately, no such miracle exists. However, exercise is the next best thing. Exercise reduces low back pain in the short term and helps prevent it in the long term. As a result, this treatment approach is consistently recommended by most guidelines for both acute and chronic low back pain, including those published by the American College of Physicians and the World Health Organization.

In the next two chapters, I will guide you step-by-step through a series of yoga poses and strengthening exercises that can help alleviate low back pain, enhance function, and prevent future painful episodes. First, it is important to understand a few basics.

A Few General Facts About Exercise

When some people think of the word *exercise,* they envision muscle-bound men and women spending hours at the gym, sweating through their spandex. If you are one of those people, let that thought go. Exercise is simply any movement made with the intention of improving health or fitness. This means exercise is *any* movement you do to help heal and prevent low back pain. No fancy clothes or expensive equipment required. Any exercise is better than no exercise at all. Starting with just a minute or two a day can make a significant difference if you do it consistently over time. The time invested in exercise not only reduces low back pain but also builds strength and confidence and can improve one's outlook on life.

Researchers have studied a wide range of exercises for low back pain—walking, running, strength training, stretching, yoga, tai chi, qigong, Pilates, and balance training—and discovered that they all work about the same. So the good news is that you can choose the exercise that best suits your preferences and lifestyle. Even better news: exercise generally requires minimal equipment or coaching. As a result, this activity is an effective low- to no-cost treatment option that fits into pretty much any schedule.

Exercise has minimal risks when done correctly. I will explain more about what "correctly" means later. The most common risk associated with exercise is mild postexercise soreness, a natural consequence of asking the body to do things it is not used to doing. And unlike many other low back treatments, exercise benefits your health rather than harming it. Even better, these benefits align with the Whole Health domains you learned about in chapter 6 and address many of the Back Factors introduced in chapter 4. Examples include improved overall wellness, better sleep, increased energy levels, and weight loss. When it comes to mental health, exercising helps with stress, anxiety, and depression. It can even decrease fear avoidance and ONTs while also increasing confidence and optimism. And because exercise can be done in groups, ranging from a walk with a friend to tens of thousands of people running a marathon together, it can also help build a sense of community and belonging. Remember, you are not alone on this journey.

What's the Catch?

With all the benefits of exercise, you knew there had to be a catch. Exercise only works if you actually do it. The same studies that show the benefits of exercise also show that most people struggle to exercise consistently over the long term. There are lots of reasons why. Finding the time can seem overwhelming. Staying motivated can be difficult. For people living with low back pain, there is also often a perceived fear of injury or worry about making the pain worse. These are legitimate obstacles. However, each can be overcome.

Remember what you learned in chapter 7: Self-empowerment is knowing what you are capable of accomplishing. Resilience is the ability to persevere even when life gets hard. Sustained motivation is doing things consistently over time, even though there are many times when you don't want to. Think about it as a continuous feedback loop. Sticking to a long-term exercise program requires self-empowerment, resilience, and sustained motivation. However, you also experience deeper levels of self-empowerment, resilience, and motivation through regular exercise. The important thing is to start where you are and make steady progress. This is possible, regardless of how little you are moving now.

For an example of how this can work, I want to introduce you to Robert. Robert and I played together as children but then lost touch until recently. Robert is sixty-two years old and has had low back pain for more than twenty-five years. When I first reconnected with Robert, he had been on total disability for the past decade, was taking opioids every day, and spent most of his time in a recliner. He mainly got up to let the dog out or use the restroom. He left his house only to go to his several doctors' appointments every month. Robert wanted more out of his life than the current status quo. I introduced him to the Whole Health approach to healing low back pain.

One of Robert's primary goals after taking the Personal Health Inventory was to walk his dog for thirty minutes every day. This would be a significant change given his sedentary lifestyle. Getting up the next morning and trying to walk a mile was not the path to success. Robert needed to move toward this goal slowly but surely. First, he ordered a step tracker online. Next, he began tracking the number of steps he usually took each day. He did this for about a week and discovered that his average daily step count was approximately 250. He decided to try walking twenty-five more steps each day and to work with a health coach on Zoom every other week. In ten days, he was walking twice as many steps. Within a month, he was walking more than 1,500 steps a day. He began taking ten-minute walks with his dog.

Three months later, Robert had met his goal of walking his dog for thirty minutes every day for the last two weeks. But that wasn't all. He also found that he was spending more time preparing healthy meals rather than eating processed food. He quit smoking. He lost twenty pounds. He worked with his primary care physician to cut the number of painkillers he was taking daily in half. He read Dr. Hazard's book, *Talking Back: How to Overcome Chronic Back Pain and Rebuild Your Life*, from cover to cover and took lots of notes. Robert experienced ups and downs during his low back pain journey. Other health issues slowed his progress at times. Early on, he sprained his ankle while walking. Robert's low back still hurts. But, he learned, it does not hurt any more than it did when he was spending his days in the recliner. And as time goes on, Robert spends far less of his time thinking about how much his back hurts. He has more energy than he has had for many years, and there are too many other things to think about that are more productive and enjoyable.

Why was Robert successful? There were several reasons. He had a clear SMART goal that was important to him. His health coach helped him stay motivated. His initial success in walking farther each day was self-empowering. This led him to wonder what else he might be capable of doing. Robert began to realize that there were many things he could do despite his pain. He felt more alert after taking fewer painkillers, which encouraged him to socialize more. He took his daughter out to dinner to celebrate her birthday and began attending church on Sunday mornings with his mother. Getting out in the world helped Robert feel more connected to other people. His small but steady string of successes led him to persevere: to keep walking every day, to keep moving, to reduce his medication use, and to expand his social life. All without ever setting foot in the gym.

The bottom line: Start where you are. Make small incremental changes. Stay focused on consistently moving in the right direction. Recognize that your daily improvements might be minor at first. However, you will be surprised at how quickly your body adapts to your new activity level, becoming stronger in the process. If you want to find out how quickly your body adapts, consider tracking your progress, as Robert did. You can use a smartwatch or a movement tracker, or simply check exercise off your to-do list every day.

If you find starting or sticking with an exercise program to be difficult, pull out the obstacle list you created in chapter 7. Add any exercise-related obstacles to the list. Next, identify the strengths you will draw upon to overcome those obstacles.

How Does Exercise Heal and Reduce Pain?

I can't think of anyone better qualified to explain the complexities of the answer to this question than Kathleen Sluka, PT, PhD. Dr. Sluka is a professor of physical therapy and rehabilitation science at the University of Iowa, where she studies causes and treatments for chronic musculoskeletal pain. As she explained to me, "Any type of exercise, such as walking or strength training, can help decrease pain. Exercise reduces pain by affecting several body systems at once, so you don't need to focus only on the painful area. When you have chronic pain, your central nervous system becomes overactive. This situation leaves the body unable to manage pain optimally. Exercise helps by increasing the body's natural painkillers, such as endorphins and serotonin, and reducing the activity of overactive neurons. In other words, exercise calms the nervous system down, so you experience less pain."

Exercise also affects the immune system. In painful conditions, the immune system releases chemicals called cytokines. Some cytokines cause inflammation and pain, while others reduce them. Regular exercise alters the immune system by reducing the cytokines that produce pain and increasing the cytokines that reduce it.

I touched briefly on systemic inflammation and it's link to diet in chapter 6. Systemic inflammation is also linked to exercise. Your immune system is highly moldable and can change based on different life circumstances. When your immune cells are stressed, they produce chemicals that can cause inflammation and pain. However, the reverse happens with regular exercise—there are increases in the chemicals that reduce pain. In addition, exercise will strengthen your body, making it easier to participate in everyday activities, from doing the laundry to walking the dog or playing with your children.

Dr. Sluka's advice when it comes to exercise? "Starting to exercise can be hard," she says, "especially for people with chronic pain. The best approach is to start small and then gradually increase activity levels."

Do the Right Exercise. Do the Exercise Right.

While some exercise is almost always beneficial for low back pain, there are two caveats: Do the right exercise. Do the exercise right.

Do the Right Exercise

I already told you that pretty much any exercise can help alleviate low back pain. Having so many choices is both an opportunity and a challenge. An opportunity because you can pick something that you really enjoy or is easy to fit into your already established routines. Challenging because it can be difficult to know where to start when you have so many choices. If you are in the challenging camp, consider beginning your exercise program by focusing on increasing your core strength, stability, and flexibility. This will help you create a strong foundation before progressing to more dynamic exercises. Core strength refers to the ability to utilize the muscles in your low back and abdominal area to move the body from one position to another. Core stability helps you maintain a steady spine, allowing you to make only the movements you choose. *Core flexibility* enhances range of motion and decreases muscle stiffness. While many people think the primary goal of exercise for the low back is to build core strength, building core stability and flexibility are equally important. A strong, stable, flexible core can help both heal and prevent low back pain. While the core is often equated with abdominal muscles, it encompasses more than just those muscles. The core also includes the muscles at the base of the pelvis and the back extensors. Hip flexors and the muscles in the buttocks (called the gluteal muscles, or "glutes") also contribute to core strength and stability.

Save high-impact exercises, such as running or jumping, and exercises that require quick movement, like tennis or pickleball, until you have worked on your core first. High-impact activities are a lot of fun and can also help prevent low back pain in the long term. However, if you are in pain now, they can also make that pain worse in the short term.

Do the Exercise Right

Exercise is a series of coordinated movements with a specific wellness goal in mind, for example, decreasing or eliminating low back pain. But remember, exercises are only helpful if they are done correctly. Each exercise includes a series of specific, sometimes subtle, movements. These movements will be covered in detail for each exercise described in chapters 9 and 10. Here are a few basics to consider first.

1. **Warm up for a few minutes before starting your exercise routine.**

   It doesn't matter what you do—walk, do a few stretches, or engage in other light movements for at least 5 minutes. If exercise is new to you, these warm-up exercises may be all you do for the first week or two. A warm-up routine puts your muscles on notice and prepares them for the work ahead.

2. **Focus on form.**

   Contracting your core muscle groups, sometimes referred to as bracing, and maintaining a relaxed, neutral spine position while exercising helps ensure you are moving correctly. This focus optimizes the impact of exercise and protects against injury.

3. **Keep your movements slow and controlled.**

   Quick movements are less helpful in building strength and more likely to lead to injury.

4. **Breathe!**

   A common mistake people make when they first start exercising is holding their breath. I know I did. Don't do that! Breathing ensures that your muscles, heart, and lungs have the oxygen they need to function properly while you are working out. Like your body movements, your breathing should be slow and controlled.

5. **Avoid overdoing it.**

   Eager to commit to a new routine, many people try to do too much too fast. Start simple. Establish a daily routine that incorporates a few exercises to enhance your core stability, strength, and flexibility and then move forward from there. A consistent routine helps create a strong foundation to build on as you progress.

You Don't Need to Exercise Alone

If exercise is new to you, consider getting help as you begin. There are numerous options, including group exercise programs at the local gym, individualized instruction, or online apps. Individualized instruction may be the best approach if you have low back pain and are new to exercise. Most physical therapists and many chiropractors provide exercise advice and instruction. Certified personal trainers and yoga instructors experienced in working with individuals with low back pain are also an option. These trained professionals can help you develop your exercise program and adjust it over time as you grow stronger and more flexible. They can also help you work on your form. Finally, they can help you stay motivated over the long term. You will find more information on how to choose the right person to help with your exercise routine in part 3 of this book.

If you would like some help but a trained professional does not work with your lifestyle or budget, there are also many good online sources of information. Focus on finding sources of information that provide insight into exercising safely and offer step-by-step instructions for a wide range of exercise options. I found the Peloton app to be a good fit for my needs, but there are many other options available.

What If Your Low Back Starts to Hurt While You Are Exercising?

If you are exercising and start to experience pain, pay attention to what your body is telling you. The appropriate action to take depends on the type of pain. If you experience some back tightness or soreness, especially a day or two after exercising, this is normal. Heat, ice, or over-the-counter NSAIDs are probably all that you need. Don't let mild discomfort keep you from exercising!

Sharp pain or significantly worse pain could be a sign of a new injury or an exacerbation of an old one. Stop what you are doing and take a few deep breaths. If the pain subsides, try the movement again more slowly. If you are fine, keep going. If the sharp pain persists, stop exercising. Otherwise, continue moving as much as possible. Heat, ice, or over-the-counter ibuprofen are likely all you'll need. If the pain persists for more than a day or two, consider scheduling an appointment with your physical therapist or chiropractor. You might also want to consult a personal trainer or someone else who specializes in exercises for people with low back pain.

Minor setbacks are to be expected when you begin a new exercise program. These setbacks are more common when other Back Factors are present, such as anxiety, stress, or prolonged periods of sitting or standing at work. Before stopping your exercise routine in response to a setback, consider making temporary adjustments to keep moving. One of the worst mistakes you can make when it comes to healing low back pain is to stop moving entirely.

Here are some modifications to consider.

- **Recheck your form** to ensure you have a neutral spine and are bracing your core correctly while moving.

- Spend a little bit more time with your **warm-up exercises.**
- Pay attention to your **breathing.**
- **Decrease** your repetitions or the weight you are using.
- See if there are **other exercises** you can do that target the same muscle groups without causing pain.
- **Don't give up!**

Now that you have a handle on the basics of exercise for low back pain, you're ready to move forward. In the next two chapters, I will introduce you to a few yoga poses and strengthening exercises so you can apply what you have learned.

Key Takeaways

- Exercise is one of the most helpful things you can do for low back pain, whether you have had low back pain for thirty minutes or thirty years.
- Starting with even a minute or two of exercise can lead to significant improvements in pain and function over time.
- It is important to do the right exercises in the right way. Get help from a trained professional if you need it.
- Movement and exercise are beneficial only as long as you engage in them regularly.
- The movement or exercise that works best for low back pain is the one that you do consistently.

chapter 9

Yoga Poses

In chapter 8, you learned why exercise is essential for managing low back pain, in addition to improving your overall health and well-being. Now it's time to focus on specific exercises to increase strength, core stabilization, and flexibility. One downside of having numerous exercise options is that it can be challenging to decide where to begin. The goal of this chapter and the next is to help you with that indecision by providing a few poses and positions to consider trying. This list is not prescriptive. Instead, think of it as a starting point.

Next you will find instructions for performing seven common yoga poses, accompanied by pictures demonstrating proper form for each pose. Most of these exercises require no more than your determination and a yoga mat.

Yoga is especially helpful in building the foundation for proper breathing and balance, preparing you for more demanding exercises. These yoga poses do not need to be done in any particular order, though you may want to end by relaxing with Savasana. First, I would like to say a few words about yoga breathing.

Yoga Breathing

Breathing correctly is a core part of any exercise routine because it helps with stability and focus as you go through the movements. In yoga, this technique is sometimes called diaphragmatic or belly breathing. Here is a quick exercise to practice belly breathing. Sit comfortably in a chair. Place your hands on your belly. Notice how your hands move as you breathe in and out at your natural rhythm. Then, when you are ready, gently inhale through your nose, drawing the breath deep into your belly. You should feel your hands move outward as you do so. Then slowly exhale through your mouth, feeling your hands and belly move inward toward your spine. Repeat. If you can't feel your belly moving when you breathe in and out, try gently pushing your belly outward into your hands when you inhale to get the process started. This can feel awkward at first, but it will come naturally with practice. Focus on breathing in and out evenly throughout each yoga position, rather than concentrating on when to inhale or exhale. Use the inhale to create length in your spine and the exhale to firm and ground your body.

Child's Pose

Targets the Spine and Lower Back

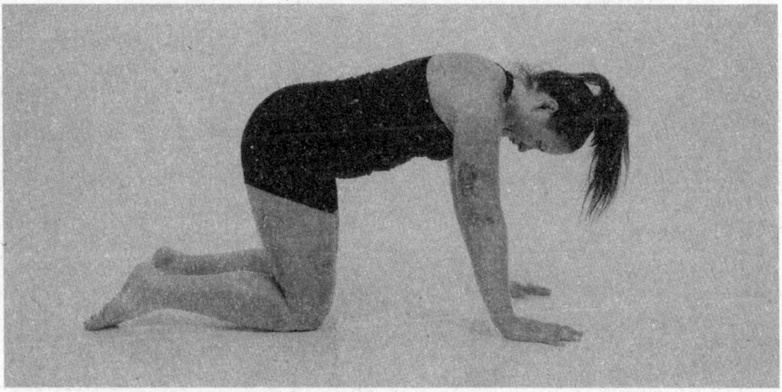

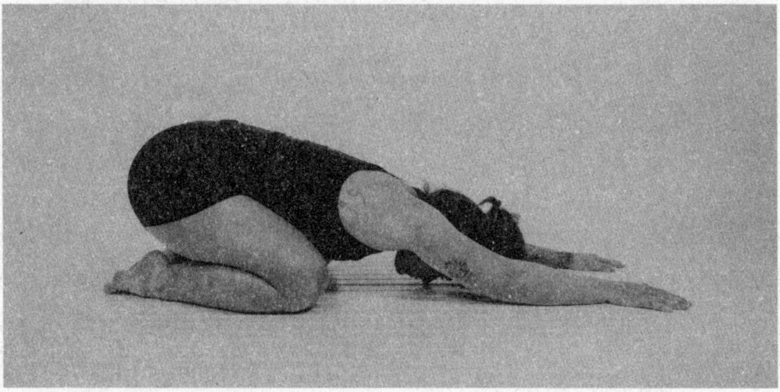

1. Start on the mat on hands and knees with your hands directly below your shoulders and your knees directly below your hips. Look straight down toward the mat. This is sometimes referred to as the tabletop position and is the starting position for several yoga poses.

2. Move your knees wider apart, approximately shoulder-width distance.

3. Point your toes toward each other.

4. Walk your hands forward about 4 to 6 inches out in front of your shoulders.

5. Push your hands down on the mat and slide them forward as you move your hips back toward your heels. Move your hips as far back as they can comfortably go. If you can touch your hips to your heels, do so.

6. Continue to push your hands down and forward.

7. As you are comfortable, bring your forehead to rest on either the floor or a block.

8. With each exhale, push your hands down and forward so that your hips settle back toward your heels. Focus on lengthening the spine while inhaling and then move the hips back toward the heels while exhaling.

9. Stay in this position for between 5 and 10 full breaths.

   Note: *The length of time you spend holding the pose should depend on how comfortable it is—if it is comfortable, remain in the pose for 10 breaths. If it feels tight or uncomfortable, begin by aiming for 5 breaths.*

10. To leave the pose, walk your hands back until they are just in front of your shoulders. Squeeze your shoulder blades together. Pull your belly in toward your spine. Push your hands down into the ground, bringing your head, shoulders, and hips up, away from your heels, and return to your hands and knees.

Cat/Cow

Targets Spinal Flexibility

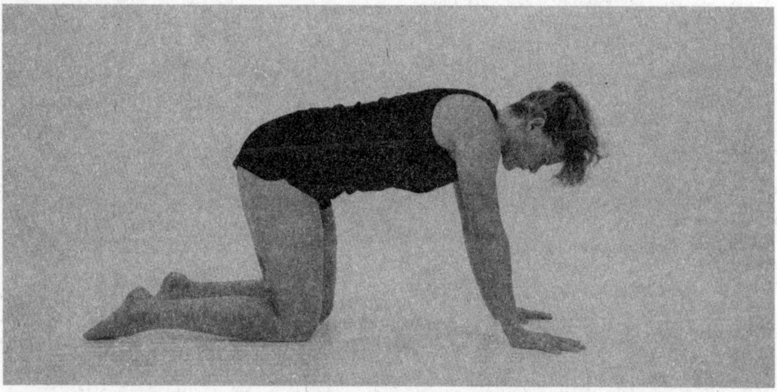

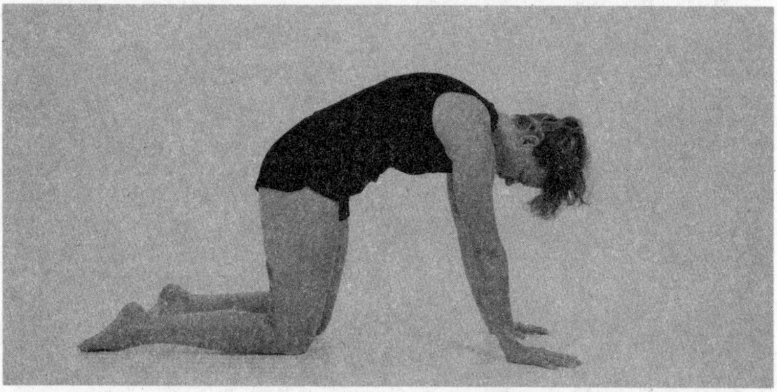

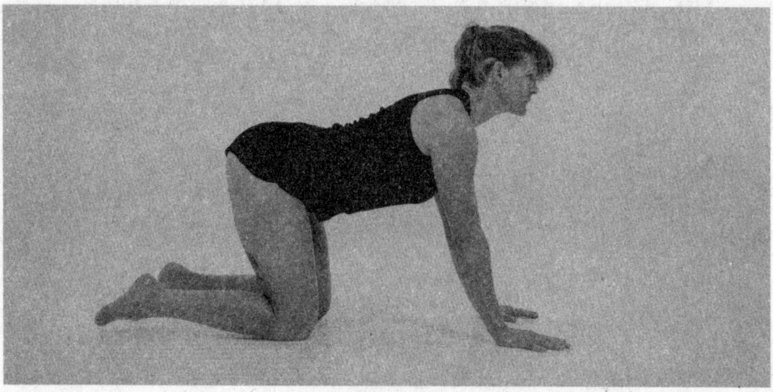

1. Start on your hands and knees on the mat, with your hands directly below your shoulders and your knees directly below your hips. Look straight down toward the mat. This is the same tabletop position you started with for child's pose.
2. Pull your belly in toward your spine.
3. Tighten your glutes.
4. Maintaining the pull, tilt your sitting bones (the bones you can feel on either side of your buttocks while sitting) upward as you pull your chin forward.
5. Lift your chin as you squeeze your shoulder blades together.
6. Your back should begin to curve into the shape of a hammock or a banana.
7. Keep pulling the belly in.
8. Hold for several breaths, feeling the stretch and your breath moving in and out.
9. Now do the opposite action. Continue to pull your hands toward your knees and your knees toward your hands, but now pretend that your rib cage is wrapped around a balloon.
10. Round and float your rib cage up toward the ceiling. Keep the belly pulling in toward the spine.
11. Drop your head, tuck your pelvis, and look in toward your thighs. Keep your glute muscles engaged.
12. Remember to keep your hands and knees pulling toward each other.
13. Unfurl and go in the opposite direction, back to the hammock/banana position. Then once again lift your rib cage toward the ceiling.

14. This is 1 rep. Begin by slowly repeating this movement back and forth, for 2 sets of 10 reps.

15. Continue to breathe evenly through the entire experience.

Easier alternative: **If this is too difficult, try standing cat/cow.**

1. Stand up straight on your mat, with your feet shoulder width apart.

2. Engage your core and tighten your glutes. Raise your hands over your head.

3. Allow your back to arch by pulling your sitting bones down and your shoulders back.

4. Bring your arms up as high as they will go, first toward the ceiling and then back behind your head.

5. Your back should be in the banana position. Hold that position for a few moments.

6. As you exhale, move in the opposite direction.

7. Bring your chin to your chest and bring your arms forward until they reach your sides, rounding your shoulders and your back around the imaginary balloon as you do so.

8. Hold that position for a few moments, then slowly and smoothly move back and forth between the banana and the balloon positions.

Bird Dog

Targets Core Stability and Balance

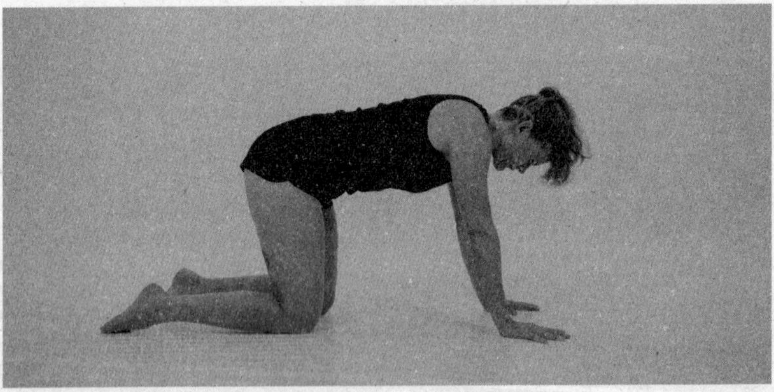

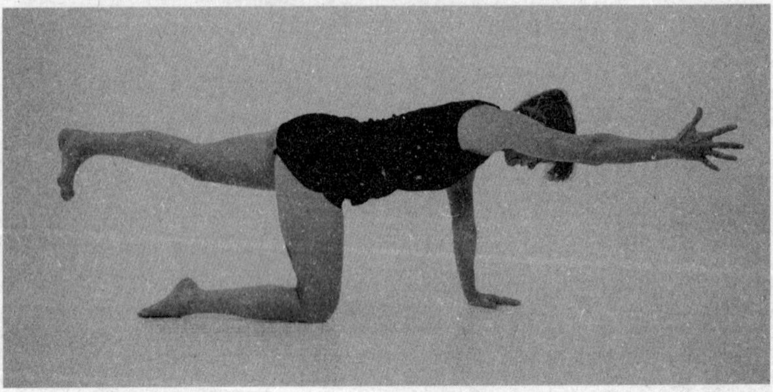

1. Start on the mat in hands-and-knees position with your hands directly below your shoulders and your knees directly below your hips. Look straight down toward the mat. Once again, this is the tabletop position.

2. Stretch your right toes back behind you on the mat. Tighten the muscles of your hip, thigh, and leg, and slowly extend your right leg until it is straight behind you.

3. Squeeze your right glute muscles.

4. Keep engaging the muscles of the right leg, all the way from your rear end down to your toes.
5. Now gently squeeze both of your legs in toward each other, so that you are engaging your inner thighs on both legs. Imagine you are holding a block between your thighs.
6. Hold this position while you walk your left fingertips out in front of you and squeeze both arms in toward each other to activate the arm muscles. Keep the right hand directly underneath your shoulder as you do this.
7. Slowly extend your left arm, reaching upward from your back, stretching the arm out away from your body.
8. Squeeze the arm muscles tight from the middle of your back, through your shoulder, to your hand.
9. Gently squeeze both legs in toward each other (again as if you were holding a block between your thighs) and both arms in toward each other, arm muscles fully engaged.
10. Hold for 2–5 complete breaths.
11. Bring your right leg and left arm back to your starting position.
12. Repeat the pose using the opposite leg and arm.
13. This is 1 rep. Repeat 3–5 times.

    Note: *Extend your arm and leg out to opposite walls with each inhale and squeeze them in closer to your center with each exhale.*

Easier alternative:

If this is too difficult or causes discomfort try separating the arm and leg exercises.

1. Begin on the mat with your hands and knees positioned directly below your shoulders and hips, respectively.
2. Look straight down toward the mat.
3. Lift and stretch your right leg toward the wall as instructed above. Hold the stretch for 2–3 breaths.
4. Bring your right leg back to the center.
5. Stretch your left arm toward the wall as instructed above. Hold the stretch for 2–5 breaths.
6. Repeat using the opposite leg and arm.
7. This is 1 rep. Repeat the entire sequence 3–5 times.

More challenging alternative:

To make this more challenging, trace small squares in the air with both your arm and leg while they are extended.

Sphinx Pose

Targets the Spine, Chest, and Lungs

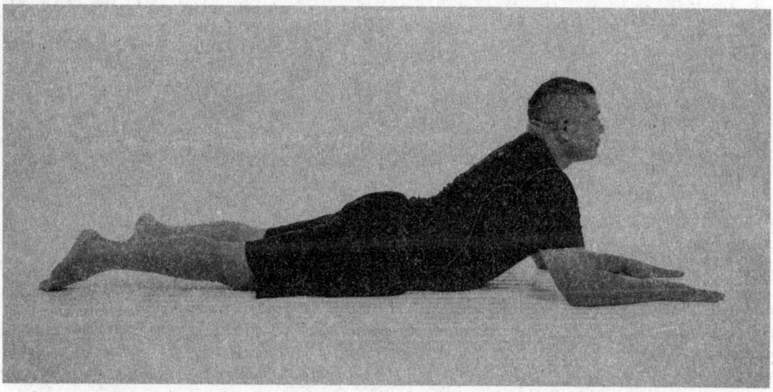

1. Lie face down on your mat with your belly facing the floor.
2. Reach your arms out in front of you, and slide/shimmy your rib cage forward so that you're lengthening your core area as much as you can.
3. Squeeze your glute muscles and hug your belly muscles in toward your spine.
4. Walk your palms back so that your hands come closer to your shoulders, with your elbows bent, propping yourself up onto your elbows. If it feels too intense on the lower back, move your elbows forward a bit more.
5. Keeping your elbows on the ground, pull them backward toward your hips, almost as though you're trying to drag yourself forward.
6. Lift your chest and your chin as you squeeze your shoulder blades together.
7. Come up as far as you can without straining your low back. How far you can come up will depend on several factors, including the level of pain you are currently experiencing.

8. Keep your belly muscles firm throughout the pose.

9. Hold this position for 2–3 breaths. Repeat 3–5 times.

10. To exit the pose, walk your arms forward again and rest your forehead on your forearms for a full inhale and exhale. Then roll over to one side, bring your knees in, and press yourself upright with your hands.

Easier alternative: **If this is too difficult or causes low back pain.**

1. Lie face down on your mat.

2. Reach your arms out in front of you and walk your rib cage forward so that you're lengthening your core area as much as you can.

3. Without propping yourself up, squeeze your glute muscles and pull your belly in tight toward your spine. Envision lengthening your entire body along the floor as much as possible, within your comfort zone.

4. Hold this position for 2–3 breaths. Repeat 5 times.

More challenging alternative:

1. To progress this pose, walk your elbows towards your shoulders until your upper arms are vertical. Your elbows will be positioned directly under your shoulders, with your forearms parallel to each other.

2. Drag yourself forward, using the pull of your elbows toward your hips and the pull of your shoulder blades toward your hips.

3. Hold this position for 2–3 breaths. Repeat 5 times.

Bridge Pose

Targets the Back, Glutes, and Hamstrings

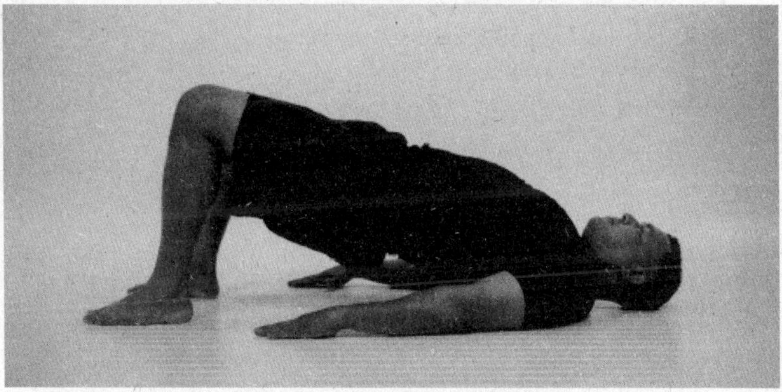

1. Lie flat on your back, face up, on your mat.
2. Bend your knees and put your feet flat on the floor or mat, keeping your feet hip width apart.
3. Place your your arms alongside your body with your elbows straight and your hands palm-side down on the floor.
4. Lift your hips and chest, keeping your feet on the ground.
5. Press your heels down, squeezing your glutes so that they lift away from the floor.
6. Press the back of your head, arms, and shoulders down into the mat.
7. Pull your belly in toward your spine. You should feel a stretch

in the front of your hips. Try to lift your hips as high as possible.

8. Stay in this position for 3–5 breaths and then lower yourself back down on the mat.

9. This is 1 rep. Repeat 3–5 times.

Eye of the Needle Pose

Targets the Outer Hips and Lower Back

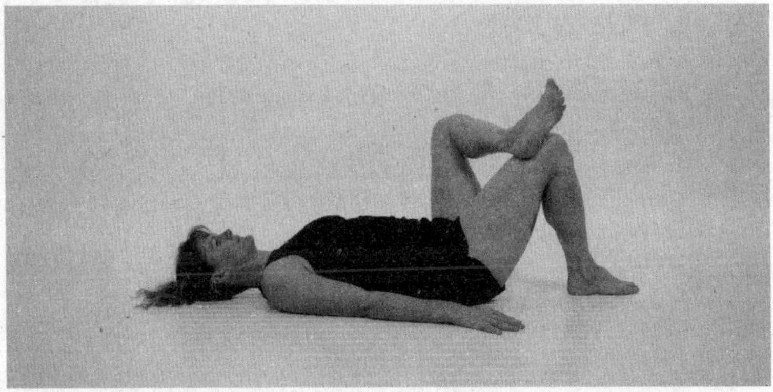

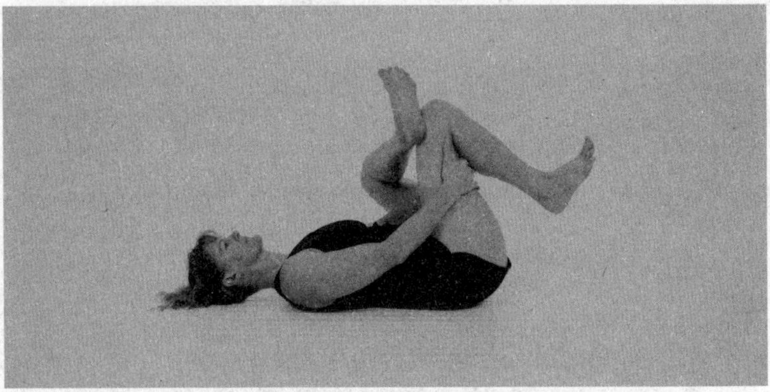

1. Lie flat on your back, face up, on your mat.
2. Place your right ankle on your left knee.
3. Turn your right leg out to the right, so that your leg is in the shape of a figure 4.
4. Flex your right foot.
5. Thread your left arm between your legs and reach around with your right arm and gently pull your left knee up toward your head.

6. Keep turning your right hip and leg outward as far as you can, feeling the muscles of your hip working as you turn the right leg out to the side.
7. Tighten your glute muscles on both sides.
8. Hold for 3–5 breaths.
9. Keep pulling the belly in toward the spine.
10. Relax back into the mat.
11. Repeat on the opposite side.
12. This is 1 rep. Repeat 3–5 times.

Easier alternative:

If this is too difficult or causes discomfort try making the pose easier.

1. Lie down on your mat, face up, bending your knees toward your chest.
2. Use your hands to push both thighs away from you. You should feel your core area lengthening as you perform this exercise.

More challenging alternative:

1. Once both legs are pulled in toward your belly, release your hands and wrap your arms around the shin of the figure-4 leg, creating a cradle for the shin as you pull it toward you.
2. Straighten the other leg away from your head toward the floor and recline back.

Savasana

Creates Balance of the Mind and Body

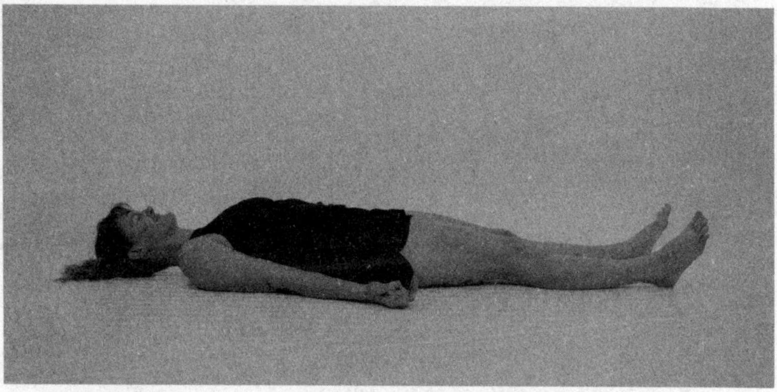

1. Lie flat on your back, face up, on your mat.
2. Straighten your legs as they rest on the mat and imagine that somebody is gently tugging your ankles away from your hips and that you are letting that happen. Reach your arms above your head and stretch for a moment or two in the same way you just did with your legs.
3. Tuck your shoulder blades underneath your body and bring your arms to your sides, palms face up.
4. Imagine your entire body is sinking into your mat.
5. Rest in this position and engage in your favorite mindfulness meditation exercise for at least 5 minutes. See chapter 13 for more information about mindfulness meditation.
6. To leave this position, turn onto one side, inhale, exhale, and then push up slowly with your palms, lifting your head last as you sit up.

Easier alternative: **If this pose causes discomfort try making the it easier.**

1. Lie down on your back with your face up, but bend your knees while keeping your feet flat on the mat.
2. Let your knees gently fall in toward each other. Arms should be positioned alongside the body, with the shoulder blades tucked underneath, and the palms facing up.
3. Let your head relax into the mat, and your knees rest against each other.
4. Hold this pose for 3 minutes if you can. Your exhales should be longer than your inhales. You can do this by inhaling for a count of 4 and exhaling for a count of 7.

Not sure if yoga is for you? You may change your mind after you hear Valerie's story.

Valerie is a sixty-seven-year-old retired schoolteacher I met through Tanya, her yoga instructor. About fifteen years ago, Valerie began experiencing pain and tension in her low back that extended into her left hip.

Here is Valerie's story:

I couldn't believe how tight and painful it was. I started with my primary care doctor, who recommended physical therapy. The physical therapist recommended TENS (transcutaneous electrical nerve stimulation) and electrical muscle stimulation. The TENS helped a little, but I was still in pain. I got an MRI. I visited Mount Sinai's sports medicine clinic and got the series of three injections that they recommended. Even though they told me that this makes the pain go away for many people, my back was hurting again within a month. Another pain clinic recommended a radiofrequency ablation. I would have said yes, but my insurance company said no. I'm glad that happened because I wound up searching for solutions on my own. I wasn't getting much help from the doctors, so I needed to figure it out for myself. I started seeing a chiropractor. I bought a TENS unit. I wore a lumbar support belt during physical activity. I saw a massage therapist. This combination of treatments was working for me, but I still had pain. Then I moved to Tucson and discovered yoga. Adding that one thing to what I was already doing helped tremendously. It is ironic because, over the years, my medical physicians told me "don't do this," or "don't do that." But I have learned that not moving is what exacerbates the pain. Plus, you start to feel like your body is useless. That is all in the past for me now. I built up my core stability. I put on about ten pounds of muscle. My overall balance got better. Today, I am stronger in every way. For the first time in many years, the pain really doesn't affect anything I do. That doesn't mean that I don't get a flare-up now and then. But when that happens, I have my "tool kit" ready to put into action and know from experience that the pain will resolve within a week or two.

When Valerie told me her story, I took away two important messages. The first message is that you really are the best person to manage your low back pain, regardless of whether your pain is new or something you have lived with for years. The second message is that supplementing your already established practices with additional treatment approaches, like yoga, can make a real difference in managing your pain.

After completing these exercises, you may have met your daily movement goal. Or, you may want to add strengthening exercises to your routine. You will find some examples of these exercises next in chapter 10.

Before you move on, one additional note. This chapter focuses on yoga poses rather than the broader context of yoga, as the latter falls outside the scope of this book. However, keep in mind that yoga is more than exercise. In addition to physical movement, yoga also includes breathwork and meditation. For a deeper dive into this practice, consider picking up a book on this topic, such as *The Yoga Bible*, by Christina Brown, or *Perfectly Imperfect: The Art and Soul of Yoga Practice*, by Baron Baptiste.

Key Takeaways

- You have a lot of flexibility when it comes to choosing which exercises are best for you.
- The yoga poses offered here are intended to help you get started. From there, you can take it on your own.
- Modify your yoga poses as needed to meet you where you are. It is best to start slowly and make steady progress from there.
- Correct breathing is a core part of any exercise routine. Belly breathing helps with stability and focus during yoga movements.
- Yoga is an excellent way to build core stability and strength.

chapter 10

Strengthening Exercises

To help get you motivated as you start your new strengthening exercise routine, I'd like you to meet Susan. Susan is fifty-eight years old and teaches English composition to freshmen at a local community college. She had low back pain on and off for ten years. As a result of her pain, Susan found herself gradually becoming less active over time. When her son gave her a membership to the local YMCA for Christmas three years ago, she thanked him politely but felt annoyed. She had no interest in being more physically active. She couldn't. Her low back hurt. Then she told Joyce, her next-door neighbor, about the gift. Joyce went to the YMCA several times a week and invited Susan to join her. In fact, she continued to invite Susan to accompany her, even though Susan repeatedly declined. The truth was that Susan was afraid. Afraid that exercising would make her low back pain worse or that it would trigger a new episode. This had happened to her before. She was worried that she couldn't figure out how to work those complicated-looking exercise machines. This had also been true in the past. She was afraid that she might make a fool of herself as she failed to do a squat, a lunge, a dead lift, or any of the exercises she had seen fit young women do on the internet. This had not happened to her yet, but she could vividly imagine it.

After about three weeks of invitations from Joyce, Susan finally said yes. The next day, Susan found herself at the YMCA, dressed in leggings and a T-shirt, shaking the hand of Joyce's personal trainer. Susan explained that she had low back pain and needed to be careful about her movements, and that she was concerned exercising might make the pain worse. The trainer assured Susan that she had worked with many people who had low back pain and that the right exercises should alleviate her back pain, not exacerbate it. The trainer went on to explain, "Our bodies are made to run, jump, twist, bend, push, pull, and move things in all sorts of directions and at all kinds of speeds. However, if we don't move enough, or in the right ways, we start losing muscle, and our bodies stop working to their full abilities." The trainer developed a personalized exercise program for Susan to build core stability, strength, and overall flexibility. To Susan's surprise, the only equipment needed was a yoga mat and two five-pound dumbbells—no scary machines. To Susan's even greater surprise, she found that the gentle exercises she started with were challenging but within her capabilities. Over time, she discovered that the squats and lunges she had once dreaded were actually based on movements she already made every day. Squats when she got in and out of a car. Lunges when she climbed stairs or stepped off a curb. Learning to perform those movements correctly and building her strength over time led to less low back pain in both the short and long term. Six months later, Susan was in better physical shape than she had been in a long time. She no longer needed her personal trainer or Joyce's text messages to get her to the gym. She was motivated by the changes she could see in her body and in her life.

Following are instructions for nine exercises, accompanied by pictures demonstrating the proper form for each. As with the yoga poses in the previous chapter, most of these exercises require no more than your determination and a yoga mat. These exercises do not need to be done in any particular order. Just be sure to warm up first by walking around the block a couple of times or doing some gentle stretches.

Dead Bug

Targets Deep Core Muscles

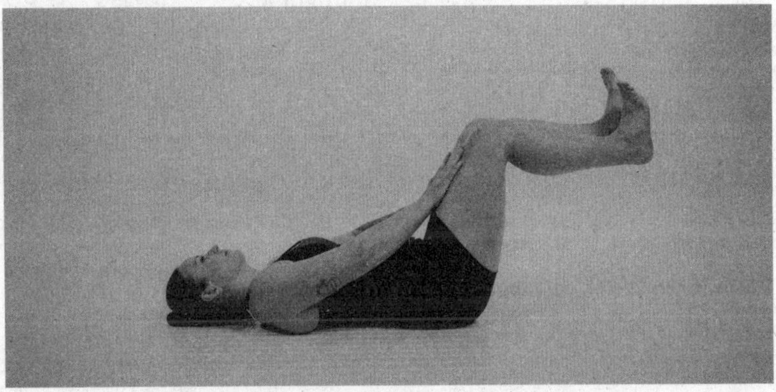

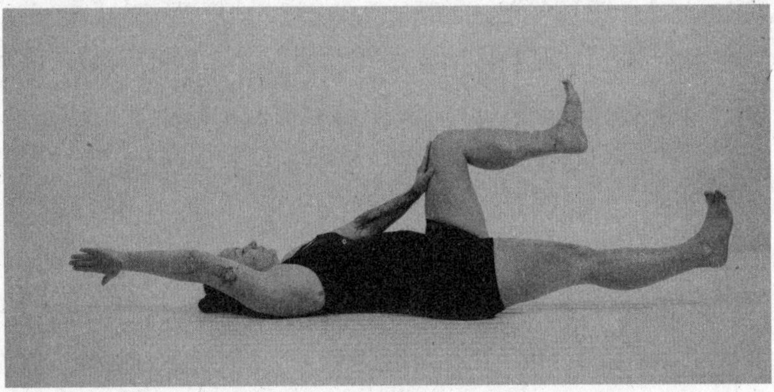

1. Lie face up with your back flat on your mat, legs extended, and arms at your sides.
2. Point your arms and legs straight up to the ceiling, legs bent 90 degrees at the knees.
3. Squeeze your glute muscles and flatten your lower back against the floor.
4. Slowly lower your right arm and your left leg at the same time, so that they are stretched out away from your body as far as you can go. Be sure to keep your low back pressed against the floor.

5. Hold this position for about 5 seconds.

6. Slowly return to center.

7. Repeat with the left arm and right leg.

8. This is 1 rep. Start with 3–5 reps.

Note: *Slowly exhale as your arms and legs extend away from your body. Do not hold your breath. The key is to apply constant downward pressure on the ground with your lumbar area.*

Easier alternative:

1. Lie on your back with your arms and legs extended straight up to the ceiling, keeping your knees bent at 90 degrees.

2. Slowly lower your right arm and your left leg so that they are pointing at opposite walls. Keep your knees bent.

3. Repeat with the left arm and right leg.

4. Alternate from side to side for 3–5 reps.

More challenging alternative:

Hold weights (or soup cans!) in each hand while making the movements described above.

Hollow Hold

Targets Core Muscles, Hip Flexors, Glutes, and Back Muscles

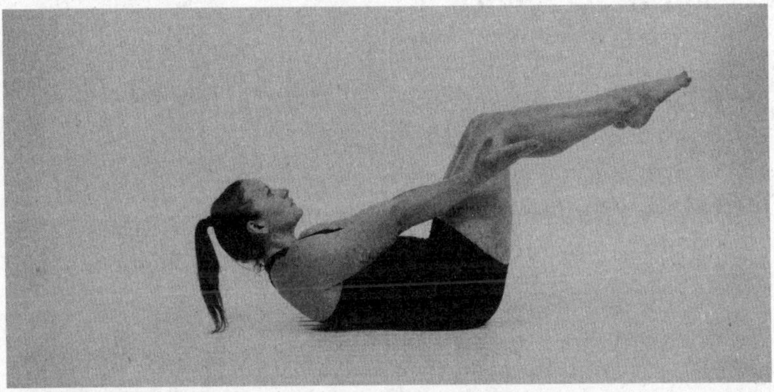

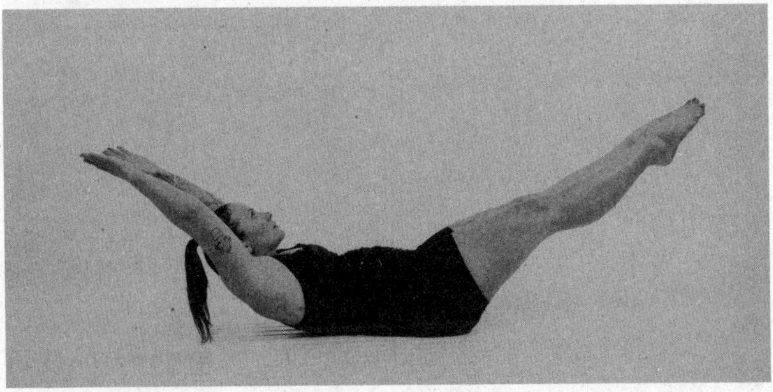

1. Lie face up with your back flat on your mat, legs extended, and arms by your sides.
2. Squeeze your glute muscles and press your low back into the mat.
3. Extend your arms over your head.
4. Look straight up toward the ceiling. Do not tuck your chin.
5. Slowly lift your feet and your shoulder blades just a few inches off the mat.

6. Hold this position while you take 2–3 slow breaths.

7. This is 1 rep. Repeat 3–5 times.

Easier alternative:

Bend your knees and reach your hands toward your toes.

More challenging alternative:

Hold the position for longer.

Knee Side Plank

Targets Deep Core Muscles and Glutes

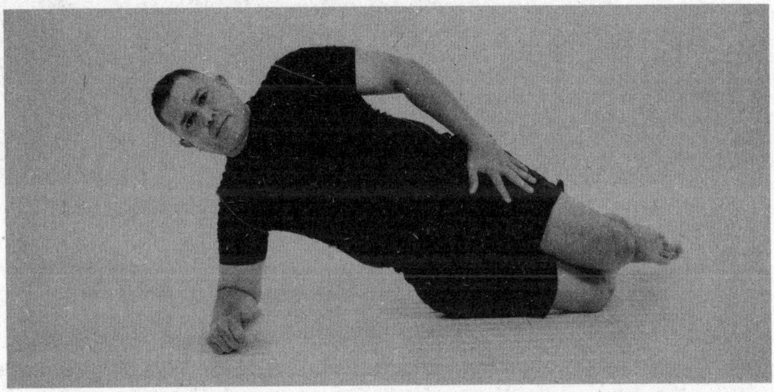

1. Lie on your right side, propped up by your right arm. Your arm should be bent at a 90-degree angle with the right elbow directly below your right shoulder.
2. Stack your hips so that the left hip is directly over your right hip.
3. Bend your knees at 90 degrees (a right angle).
4. Squeeze your glute muscles.
5. Lift your right hip off the ground.
6. Exhale as you push your body away from the mat.
7. Your ear, shoulder, hips, and knees should be in a straight line as you push yourself up.
8. Keep your shoulders in line with each other.
9. Hold for 3–5 breaths. Slowly lower yourself back to the mat.
10. Repeat on the opposite side.
11. This is 1 rep. Repeat 3–5 times.

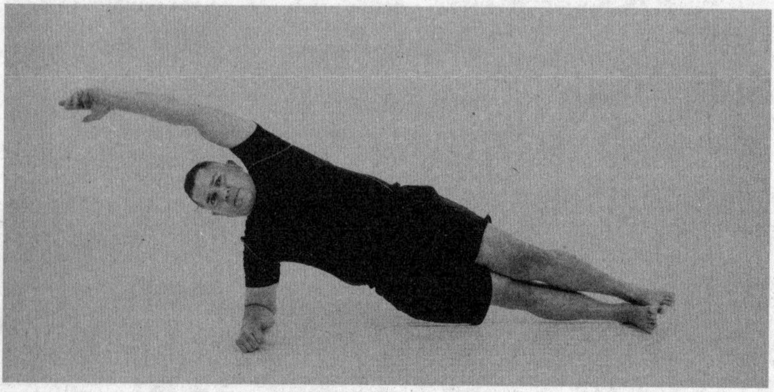

More challenging alternative:

1. Lie on your right side with your right elbow on the ground, but this time with your legs fully extended and your left foot stacked on top of your right foot.
2. Squeeze your glute muscles. Push your entire body away from the ground with your elbow, so that only your elbow and your feet are touching the ground.
3. Hold for 2–3 breaths and slowly lower yourself back down to your side.
4. Repeat on the opposite side.
5. This is 1 rep. Do 3–5 reps on each side.

Squats

Targets the Glutes, Thighs, and Core Muscles

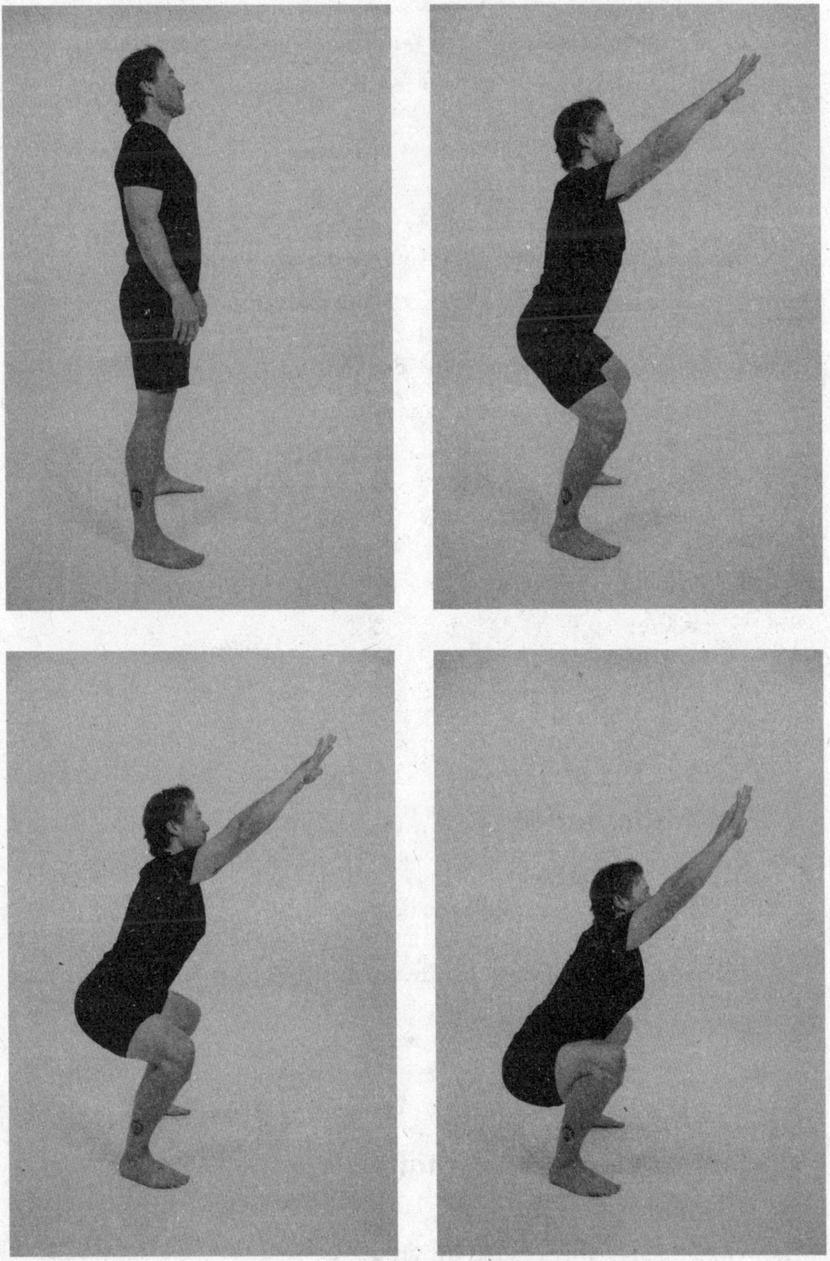

1. Stand on your mat with your feet roughly shoulder width apart and your toes pointed out slightly.

2. Bend your knees slightly and push your feet firmly into the ground.

3. Rotate your knees slightly outward to activate your glute muscles, making sure that your feet are still flat on the ground.

4. Push your hips toward the wall behind you as if you were sitting down in a chair.

5. Bend your knees and lower yourself down toward the ground as far as you can go comfortably. Keep your chest up and your back straight.

6. Start with your hands extended in front of you at shoulder height and raise them up as you squat down to help maintain a straight back.

7. Hold this position for 2–3 breaths.

8. Push into the mat with your feet as you return to a standing position.

9. This is 1 rep. Repeat 3–5 times.

Easier alternative:

1. Stand with your back to a chair.

2. Squat until your butt lightly touches the chair.

3. Return to a standing position.

More challenging alternative:

Lower yourself farther toward the ground.

Lunges

Targets Glutes, Upper Leg, and Hip Flexor Muscles

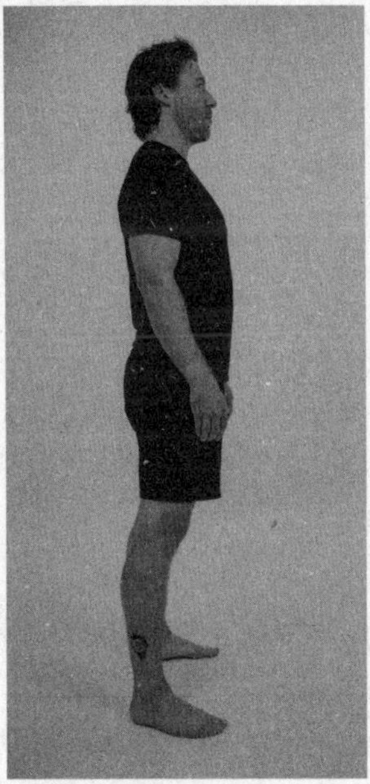

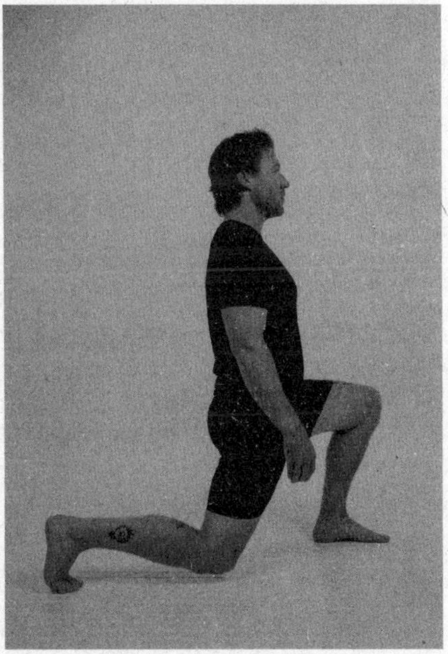

1. Stand on your mat with your feet directly under your hips.
2. Step forward with your right leg, heel first.
3. Keep your arms hanging down at your sides.
4. Bend both knees, pointing your left knee toward your mat.
5. Slowly lower your body toward your mat as far as you comfortably can.
6. Your right knee should be positioned between your ankle and your toes.
7. Your left knee should be in line with your left hip and shoulder.
8. Hold this position for 1–2 breaths.

9. Push your right heel into your mat to return to your starting position.
10. Repeat on the opposite side. Begin by stepping the left foot forward.
11. This is 1 rep. Repeat 3–5 times.

Easier alternative:

Step backward instead of forward, lower yourself only slightly toward the ground, or hold on to the side of a chair for stability.

More challenging alternative:

Lower yourself closer to the ground or step forward so that you are "walking" as you switch from one leg to the other.

Single Leg Step Up: *Targets Glutes and Thigh Muscles*

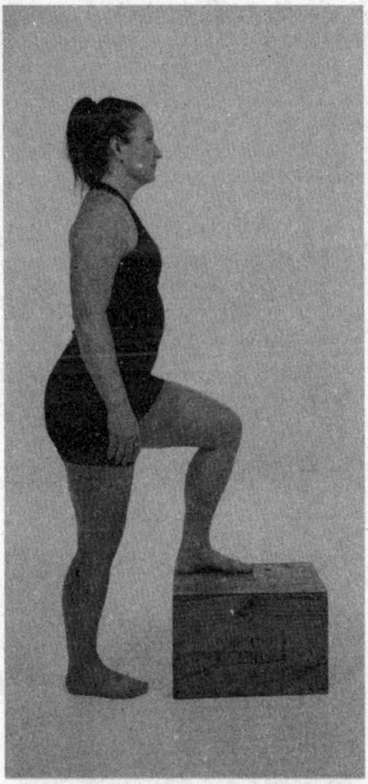

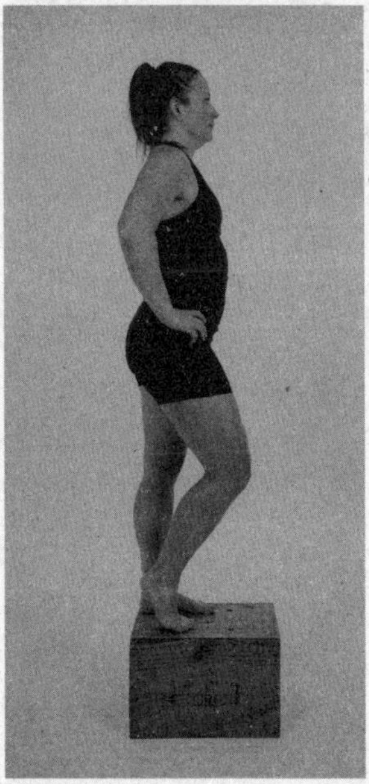

1. Stand facing a sturdy box or step.
2. Slowly place your right foot up on the step.
3. Pause for a breath or two.
4. Slowly lift your left foot onto the step, keeping your chest up and your back straight.
5. Step slowly backward onto the floor with your left foot.
6. Keep your arms down at your sides.
7. Repeat 5 times with each leg.

Easier alternative:

Use a lower step.

More challenging alternative:

Use a higher step or hold a weighed object in each hand.

Superman

Targets Glutes, Hamstrings, and Back Muscles

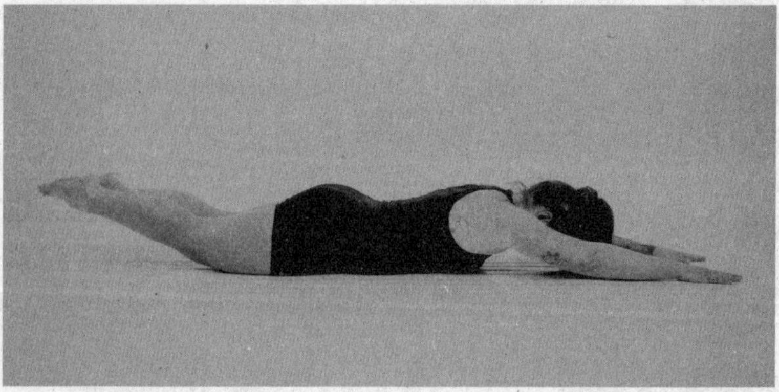

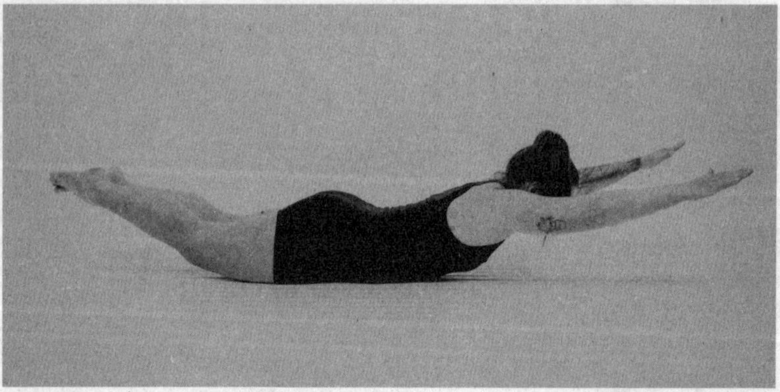

Note: *Superman strengthens your erector spinae muscles, which can help improve overall spine stability. However, this position can also make low back pain worse for some people. If you are one of those people, start with the easier alternative described below.*

1. Lie face down on your mat with your legs extended and your arms at your sides.

2. With your face still looking directly down into the mat, extend your arms forward.

3. Squeeze your glute muscles and push your belly firmly into the ground.

4. Slowly lift your arms and legs about 6 inches off the floor.

5. Your head should be even with your arms, looking down toward the ground.

6. Hold this position for 3–5 breaths.

7. Slowly lower your arms and legs back down to the mat.

8. This is 1 rep. Repeat 3–5 times.

Easier alternative:

1. Slowly raise your arms off the mat.

2. Hold for 2–3 breaths. Slowly lower your arms.

3. Slowly raise your legs about 6 inches off the mat, then lower them just as slowly.

4. Repeat 5 times.

More challenging alternative:

Hold your arms and legs off the mat for 10 breaths.

Good Mornings

Targets Hamstrings, Glutes, and Lower Back

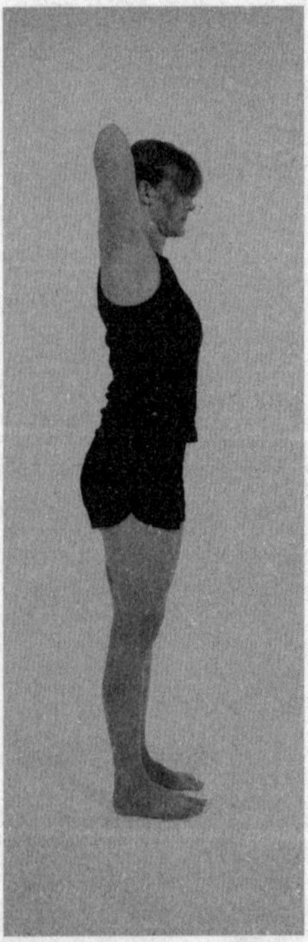

1. Stand on your mat with your feet directly under your hips.
2. Bend your knees slightly.
3. Place your hands behind your head (as if you were doing a sit-up).
4. Squeeze your glute muscles and pull your ribs down, engaging your core muscles as you do so.
5. Keep your back straight as you slowly hinge forward at the hips until your chest is parallel to your mat.
6. Hold for 2–3 breaths. Push your feet into the mat to help you return to a standing position.
7. This is 1 rep. Repeat 5 times.

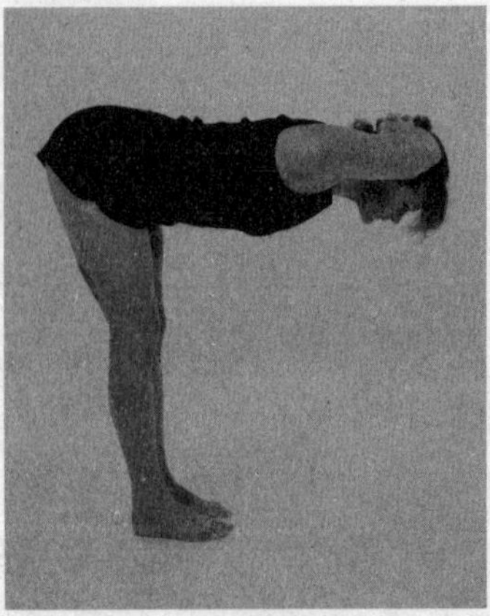

Easier alternative:

Begin in a seated position.

More challenging alternative:

Move on to a dead lift (see next page).

Dead Lift

Targets the Low Back, Glutes, and Hamstrings

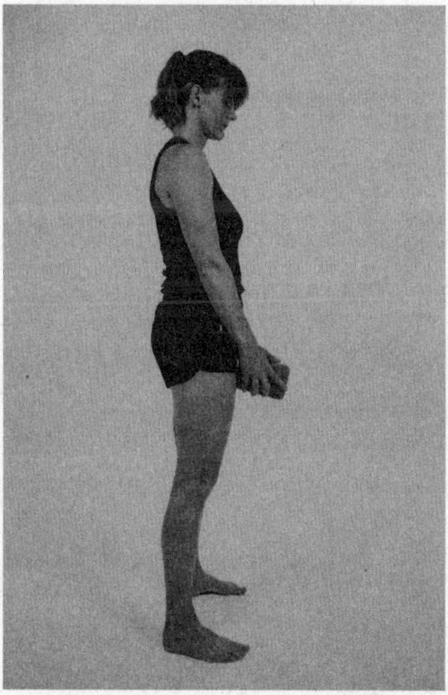

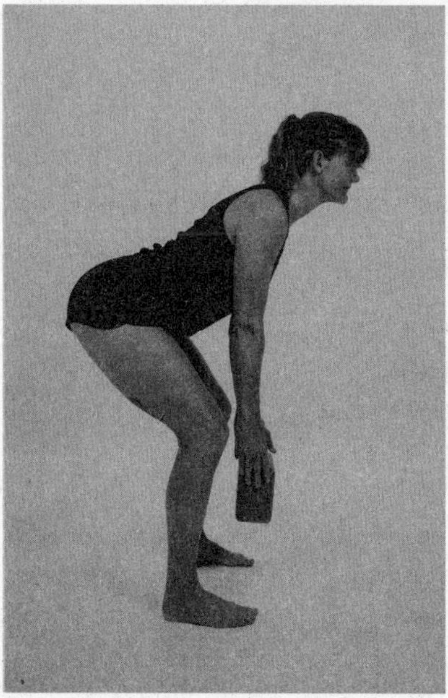

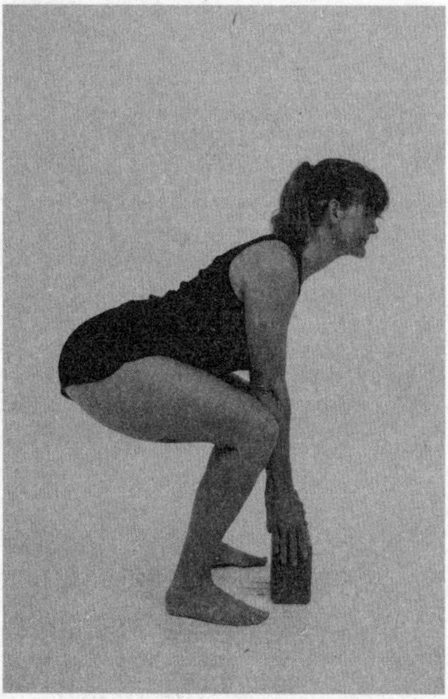

1. Place an object on the floor in front of you, between your big toes. The object can be anything you can lift comfortably, ranging from a kettlebell or yoga block to common household items such as a can of food or a bag of flour.
2. Stand on your mat with your feet directly under your hips.
3. Bend your knees slightly.
4. Rotate your shoulders back and down.
5. Squeeze your glute muscles and pull your ribs down, engaging your core muscles as you do so.
6. Keep your back straight as you slowly hinge forward at the hips until your hands are at knee height.
7. Bend your knees until your hands reach the object in front of you.
8. Keep your back straight and core tight as you push into the mat with your feet.
9. Pick the object up off the ground and return to a standing position.

Easier alternative:

Use a lighter object.

More challenging alternative:

Use a heavier object.

Once you are comfortable with these exercises, consider customizing your routine by introducing new exercises to target specific body parts or movements. If you are concerned that strengthening exercises are not for you because you are overweight or have heart disease, an inactive lifestyle, or too many things wrong with your low back, talk with your healthcare professional about starting an exercise program. But first, meet Joel for inspiration.

Joel will soon turn fifty. It is not just his low back pain that has made the last few years tough. He has high blood pressure. He thinks he is overweight. He had a hip replacement. His job as a grocery store manager is stressful. His MRI shows lumbar spondylolisthesis and spinal stenosis. Different medical physicians told him, "There is nothing we can do for you to help with the pain"; "Try gabapentin"; "Take Lyrica"; "Get a series of corticosteroid injections"; "You need spine surgery." For the first three years, Joel was frustrated, afraid to be physically active, caught in a cycle of work and home, with little time or energy for anything else. Then, two years ago, Joel's local university recruited people with cardiovascular risk factors for a research project on exercise. He signed up. When the program ended two months later, Joel realized he had less low back pain and felt a lot healthier overall. He didn't want to stop exercising. He signed up for CrossFit. "At first," he says, "I kept getting hurt because I was trying to keep up with the twenty-year-olds." Finally, he talked with his strength and conditioning coaches, Nathan and Christy. "I told them the problems I was having," he says. "They helped me modify my exercise program so that it worked for me. They emphasized the importance of good form, breathing correctly, and keeping my core tight while exercising. I still have pain, but it doesn't stop me from doing the things that are important to me. It's a balancing act. I'm not going to be a powerlifter, but I can sure do a lot of squats. And I'm stronger than I've ever been in my entire life."

During his last doctor's visit, the physician told Joel that he had so many issues going on with his low back, it should have been impossible to put in a full day's work and still be able to walk. Joel's response? "I told him that I could deadlift 315 pounds. The doctor grinned from ear to ear and told me, 'I hear what you're telling me, but it just doesn't make sense with your current spine. Keep doing what you're doing.' I thought that was a huge win."

Key Takeaways

- Once again, any exercise is better than no exercise at all.
- Susan and Joel show us that exercise can lead to significant improvements in overall health and managing low back pain.
- Exercises focused on core stability, core strength, and overall flexibility are a good way to get started.
- Modify your exercise program as needed to meet you where you are at.
- Consider working with a trained professional who is knowledgeable about both exercise and low back pain to develop a personalized plan targeting your specific needs.

chapter 11

Common Self-Care Treatments

Knowing as much as possible about your many treatment options can help guide you in the right direction during your low back pain journey. The purpose of the next several chapters is to provide you with the information you need to make informed treatment decisions. This includes which treatments have been shown to be most effective for low back pain, which ones are ineffective, and which are best for specific cases. You will also learn what researchers have discovered about each treatments' safety and which Back Factors they address.

In this chapter, you will learn about treatments commonly used for low back pain that you can easily buy for yourself or access through a healthcare professional. Examples include ice packs, superficial heat sources, and over-the-counter pain medications. The goal of these treatments is usually temporary pain relief. They are unlikely to address the underlying causes of your low back pain or your Back Factors. You will notice that low back pain guidelines from the American College of Physicians and the World Health Organization do not recommend many of these treatments. I still want to highlight them because they are generally safe, easily accessible, and effective for some individuals.

As you consider these treatments, keep in mind that there is no one-size-fits-all approach. Each therapy has a stated benefit that may or may not have been validated by research, as well as known, albeit low, risks. As with every approach you consider for your low back pain, it is essential to balance the potential benefits against the possible risks. That equation is slightly different for everyone. Adhere to the manufacturer's and/or prescribing physician's instructions when using over-the-counter medication or devices. This is especially important if you are pregnant or nursing or have other medical conditions. Also, if you have questions or experience side effects while using any of these treatment approaches, talk with your healthcare professional.

Table 11.1 provides a brief description of the treatments included in this chapter, along with a quick reference on low back pain guideline recommendations for each.

Self-Care Treatments

Table 11.1

Self-Care Treatment	Description	Low Back Pain Guideline Recommendations
Nonsteroidal anti-inflammatory drugs	Over-the-counter pain medication	Recommended by ACP and WHO
Acetaminophen	Over-the-counter pain medication	Not recommended by ACP Recommended against by WHO
Topical cayenne pepper	Applying capsaicin cream, gel, or patch to the skin over a painful area	Not addressed by ACP Recommended by WHO
Topical lidocaine or menthol	Applying medicated cream, gels, patches, or sprays to the skin over a painful area	Not addressed by ACP or WHO
Superficial heat	Applying a low-level source of heat to the skin	Recommended by ACP Not addressed by WHO
Cold therapy	Applying ice or a cold source to the skin	Not addressed by ACP or WHO
Lumbar braces and supports	Using belts or corsets to support the low back	Not addressed by ACP WHO is neutral
Orthotics	Placing inserts in the shoe	Not addressed by ACP or WHO

Self-Care Treatment	Description	Low Back Pain Guideline Recommendations
Posture and ergonomics	Body positioning and ergonomic devices	Not addressed by ACP or WHO
Electrotherapies, transcutaneous electrical nerve stimulation (TENS)	Mechanical device unit that produces weak electrical currents	Not addressed by ACP Recommended against by WHO Recommended by some European guidelines
Bed rest	Rest as a medical treatment	Recommended against by WHO Not addressed by ACP

ACP, American College of Physicians; WHO, World Health Organization.

Nonsteroidal Anti-Inflammatory Drugs

Nonsteroidal anti-inflammatory drugs, often abbreviated as NSAIDs, are available both over the counter and at prescription strength. Examples that you may be most familiar with are aspirin, ibuprofen (Advil, Midol, and Motrin), and naproxen (Aleve). NSAIDs are available in tablet, capsule, or liquid form or as a patch or gel.

How does it work?

As the name suggests, NSAIDs temporarily reduce inflammation in the body.

Is it effective?

NSAIDs can lead to short-term decreases in low back pain and improvements in physical function. As a result, this drug is widely recommended by low back pain guidelines for both acute and chronic low back pain. Of note, the ACP recommends that you consider NSAIDs after you have tried nondrug therapies, such as exercise, acupuncture, and spinal manipulation.

Is it safe?

NSAIDs are among the safest of all medications available to treat low back pain, but they still carry risk, especially for some people. Common side effects include indigestion, headaches, dizziness, and allergic reactions. More serious but rare side effects include ulcers, internal bleeding, heart attacks, and stroke. Internal bleeding caused by NSAIDs is more likely to happen in older adults, people taking higher doses of NSAIDs, people taking NSAIDs regularly for weeks or months at a time, those at risk of cardiovascular disease or stroke, and those who are taking blood thinners to prevent stroke or heart attack. NSAIDs can also make asthma worse and should be avoided by people with chronic kidney disease. Seek help immediately if you experience any signs of internal bleeding, such as extreme fatigue, unexplained bruising, or symptoms of a heart attack or stroke.

Is it easily accessible?

Over-the-counter-strength NSAIDs are available online and at drugstores and grocery stores throughout the United States, starting at a cost of around $10 for five hundred 200 mg generic capsules. Prescription-strength NSAIDs can be prescribed by medical physicians, nurse practitioners, and physician assistants.

Other considerations:

NSAIDs are widely recommended for low back pain. However, this medication should be used only for a short time, and preferably only after you have tried nondrug treatments such as spinal manipulation and acupuncture first. It is important to discuss the use of NSAIDs with your physician, especially if you are over sixty, take blood thinners, or are at risk of cardiovascular disease.

Acetaminophen

Acetaminophen is available both over the counter and at prescription strength. It is best known as Tylenol in the United States, but in most of the rest of the world, it is called paracetamol or Panadol.

How does it work?

Acetaminophen interrupts the chemical messengers in your body that tell your brain you are experiencing pain.

Is it effective?

Acetaminophen does not work better than a placebo (sugar pill) for low back pain. As a result, it is not recommended by low back pain guidelines.

Is it safe?

Acetaminophen is safer for many people than NSAIDs, but it doesn't work as well, and side effects are possible, especially for some people. The most common side effects are nausea, stomach pain, and headache, but Tylenol can also cause severe liver damage. This is primarily a concern for people who drink more than two or three alcoholic beverages per day or have known liver disease.

Is it easily accessible?

Acetaminophen is readily available in pill or liquid form at drugstores and grocery stores and online, starting at around $5 for two hundred 500 mg generic tablets.

Other considerations:

Acetaminophen is often combined with other medications, including pain relievers and certain cold and cough remedies. As a result, it is essential to read the list of ingredients in any medications you are taking to avoid taking too much of this drug.

Topical Cayenne Pepper

Topical cayenne pepper is a pain reliever available as a cream, gel, or patch. It is applied directly to the skin over the painful area. The main ingredient is capsaicin, the substance in chili peppers that causes a burning sensation when you eat them.

How does it work?

Capsaicin is thought to deplete a chemical in cells that transmits pain and heat signals, thereby interrupting pain signals to the brain.

Is it effective?

While more research is needed on topical cayenne pepper, available studies provide some evidence of effectiveness. When my colleague Dr. Erin Krebs, chief of general internal medicine at the Minneapolis VHA Health Care System, conducted a clinical trial comparing different medications for low back pain, one of her surprise findings was the number of people who reported good results when using capsaicin. The WHO recommends topical cayenne pepper for chronic low back pain.

Is it safe?

Overall, topical cayenne pepper is safe if you follow the manufacturer's instructions. The most common side effect is skin irritation at the application site. As with any medication or supplement, allergic reactions, including swelling, rash, or difficulty breathing are possible, though very rare in this case.

Is it easily accessible?

Topical cayenne pepper is available online and at some drug and health food stores, starting at around $25. Follow the manufacturer's instructions when applying cayenne pepper. Those instructions will vary depending on the type of application (cream, gel, or patch) and the capsaicin concentration.

Other considerations:

Be sure to wash your hands immediately after using topical cayenne pepper, and avoid getting it in your eyes, nose, mouth, or other sensitive areas of your body. An inconvenient aspect of this treatment approach is that it works only if the creams or gels are used regularly, usually three to four times a day.

Topical Lidocaine or Menthol

Topical pain relievers are creams, gels, patches, and sprays that you apply directly to the skin over a painful area. They are available both over the counter and at prescription strength, depending on the active ingredients. Examples (in addition to NSAIDs and cayenne pepper) are lidocaine (doses over 4 percent require a medical physician's prescription) and menthol (a substance found in peppermint oil). Topical pain relievers can be purchased as a one-substance option or in a combined form.

How does it work?

Lidocaine blocks pain signals to the brain. Menthol provides a cooling sensation that is thought to "distract" your body from the pain.

Is it effective?

There is little to no research on the use of lidocaine or menthol topical pain relievers for low back pain. However, they appear to be at least somewhat helpful for other musculoskeletal conditions, such as ankle sprains or strains.

Is it safe?

Menthol is safe. The primary side effects are redness or mild skin irritation at the application site. Lidocaine is mostly safe at the doses available over the counter. The most common risks are skin irritation or rash. However, it can be dangerous at higher doses. Signs of overdose include irregular heartbeat, seizures, and trouble breathing. Keep this product away from children and pets. Avoid using it in areas with open cuts or sores, or on covered areas, as this may increase absorption through the skin. As with any medication, allergic reactions are possible with topical pain relievers, although they are very rare.

Is it easily accessible?

Topical pain relievers are available in various forms, including creams, gels, patches, and sprays, and can be easily found at pharmacies, grocery stores, and online retailers. The cost of topical pain relievers starts at around $15.

Other considerations:

Wash your hands right after applying the lotion or gel, and avoid getting it in your eyes, nose, mouth, or other sensitive areas of the body.

Superficial Heat

Superficial heat involves applying a low-level heat source to the body.

How does it work?

Heat warms the skin and the tissues underneath, decreasing muscle stiffness and increasing flexibility. It may also block pain signals to the brain by acting on the nerve endings in your skin. In addition, heat increases blood flow in the area where it is applied, bringing fresh oxygen to the area while also removing waste materials generated by your back muscles.

Is it effective?

Superficial heat therapy can lead to temporary reductions in low back pain and improvements in physical functioning. Most guidelines for low back pain, including those published by the American College of Physicians, recommend superficial heat as a treatment option for acute and chronic low back pain.

Is it safe?

Superficial heat is generally safe, but it still carries some risks. The most common side effect of superficial heat is short-term reddening or a pinkish tone in the skin directly under the heat application. Burns can occur if your heat source is too hot. Avoid superficial heat if you have any illness that reduces your ability to feel sensations, such as diabetic neuropathy, autoimmune disorders, or multiple sclerosis. Talk with your physician before using heat if you have poor circulation or active cancer.

Is it easily accessible?

There are several types of superficial heat. A heat source, such as a hot pack, heat wrap, or heating pad, can be placed over the skin in the affected area. These heat sources are readily available at drugstores and online, starting at around $10–$15. Another option is to immerse oneself in a warm bath, hot tub, or sauna. Apply heat for 15–20 minutes at a time. Use superficial heat as needed, but not more often than once an hour.

Other considerations:

Regardless of how long you have had low back pain, superficial heat can be a good starting point. It is inexpensive, reasonably safe (if the heat source is not too hot), and easy to do on your own. Plus, for most people, it feels good while you are doing it.

Cold Therapy

Cold therapy involves applying cold or ice to the skin. The ice packs you buy in the store can contain various substances, including gel-like materials, water, and propylene glycol (a chemical that helps water freeze faster).

How does it work?

Cold therapy is thought to reduce inflammation, numb pain, and temporarily decrease swelling.

Is it effective?

The internet is full of clinical sites that recommend cold therapy for low back pain. However, researchers are less sure. Few studies exist, and most don't show a clear benefit. As a result, cold therapy is not recommended by most low back pain guidelines.

Is it safe?

Cold therapy is generally safe, but some risks are still associated with it. The most common side effect is frostbite. This can largely be avoided by ensuring that the cold source does not come into direct contact with the skin. Immersing yourself in icy water is not recommended, as it can strain your heart.

Is it easily accessible?

Making an ice pack can be as simple as freezing ice in a plastic bag or repurposing a bag of frozen vegetables. You can also buy ice packs in different sizes, shapes, and materials at any drugstore, starting at about $10. Apply ice packs, cold compresses, or ice massage to the skin over the area where your low back hurts. To prevent frostbite, avoid putting the cold source directly on your skin. Wrap the ice or cold pack in a dish towel first. Leave it on for ten to twenty minutes but no longer than twenty minutes. Apply as needed but no more often than once an hour.

Other considerations:

Despite the lack of data, there is no reason not to try cold therapy for temporary relief of low back pain. People in my household have been known to apply a bag of frozen peas to a sore back after shoveling snow or mowing the lawn. Just don't eat the peas afterward. Eating thawed and refrozen food is a classic source of food poisoning.

Lumbar Braces and Supports

Lumbar braces and supports are thick belts or corsets that are secured tightly around the body over the painful area of your lower back.

How does it work?

It is believed that limiting back muscle movement and providing additional support can help alleviate low back pain.

Is it effective?

Although there is limited research available to guide us, the available data suggest that wearing back braces and supports does not decrease pain or improve function compared to not wearing them. The guidelines that address lumbar braces and supports generally recommend against them, though the World Health Organization is neutral.

Is it safe?

Using lumbar braces and supports for extended periods can weaken and destabilize your back muscles. Some people start to depend on them, thinking that they might get hurt worse if they are not wearing the support or brace. This may lead to fear avoidance or ONTs.

Is it easily accessible?

Lumbar braces and supports are available online, at most pharmacies, and from some healthcare professionals, including medical physicians, physical therapists, and chiropractors. Costs for lumbar braces and supports start at around $25 but can quickly increase, especially if you purchase them in a healthcare professional's office.

Other considerations:

Lumbar braces and supports may be helpful temporarily if you are in extreme pain and they are able to help you stay active. However, it is incredible how quickly muscles lose strength when they are not used. Talk with your healthcare professional before using lumbar braces and supports for more than a few days.

Orthotics

Orthotics are devices inserted into your shoes. They are designed to adjust your foot position, thereby changing how you walk or hold your body. There are several different types of orthotics, but arch supports, or insoles, are typically used for low back pain.

How does it work?

Orthotics are designed to help improve posture and correct gait imbalances, thereby reducing stress on the spine. However, no research has shown explicitly that these biomechanical changes affect low back pain.

Is it effective?

More research is needed on the effectiveness of orthotics in the treatment of low back pain. Few studies are available, and the results are conflicting. It is possible that custom orthotics are more effective than those purchased over the counter.

Is it safe?

Orthotics are generally safe. However, for some people, the change in posture or gait caused by orthotics may temporarily exacerbate low back pain.

Is it easily accessible?

A wide range of insoles and arch supports is available, ranging from generic options that can be purchased at any drugstore starting at around $12. Custom-made options available through podiatrists or chiropractors tend to be more expensive.

Other considerations:

Orthotics are safe to use and can be helpful for conditions like plantar fasciitis or heel spurs. The jury is still out on their usefulness for low back pain. More research is needed.

Posture and Ergonomics

Posture refers to the way you naturally hold your body when sitting, standing, or moving about, while ergonomics relates to the positions your body must adapt to at the workplace to perform your job effectively. In addition to advice on changing your posture or ergonomic environment, numerous devices and workplace equipment modifications are available.

How does it work?

Postural change typically involves efforts to stand or sit up straight, or to adjust the curvature of your spine. Postural devices are designed to help with maintaining optimal posture. Ergonomic advice includes optimizing your workspace with chairs that fit your body and workstations that minimize strain on your back muscles.

Is it effective?

There is limited research to support the notion that maintaining proper posture when sitting or using a new desk chair at work can alleviate low back pain. While some studies suggest that posture and ergonomics are linked to low back pain, it remains unclear which comes first. These associations may have more to do with a lack of movement for extended periods than with the curvature of your spine, while proper lifting techniques may be more closely related to core stability. Low back pain guidelines do not recommend postural advice/devices and ergonomics.

Is it safe?

There are few risks associated with postural control and ergonomics. However, forcing yourself into uncomfortable postures can increase your pain.

Is it easily accessible?

Numerous resources on posture and ergonomics are available online. Some of them come from healthcare professionals. Many physical therapists and chiropractors focus on these topics. You will also find advice from companies that manufacture wearable devices that help you to stand up straight, apps that remind you to stand up straight, and adjustable desk chairs that help you sit up straight.

Other considerations:

Neither posture nor ergonomics is strongly correlated with low back pain. Instead, you may want to focus on physical activity. As Duke chiropractor Dr. Ben Holmes once told me, "When I first started treating patients, I focused a lot on posture and ergonomics. I advised patients to sit up straight and recommended consulting an ergonomic specialist to evaluate their workspaces. Over time, I realized that people did better if they moved more. Now I tell them to set their phone alarm to remind them to get up and walk around every hour."

Electrotherapies, Transcutaneous Electrical Nerve Stimulation

Transcutaneous electrical nerve stimulation, or TENS, also sometimes called a TENS unit, is a small, battery-powered device that delivers a low-level electrical impulse to your body through electrodes attached to your skin with sticky pads.

How does it work?

TENS sends electrical pulses through the skin to enhance your body's natural pain-reducing ability. The electrical pulses can release the body's natural painkillers, endorphins, and other chemicals to stop pain signals in the brain.

Is it effective?

Based on current research, the effectiveness of TENS for treating low back pain remains unclear. However, Dr. Sluka, whom you met in chapter 8, believes that most TENS studies on low back pain did not use appropriate research methods, as researchers ignored important issues related to the practical application of the unit in real-world settings. Her studies show that TENS produces the largest benefit while people are engaged in movement. She has also learned that TENS reduces pain only while the device is actually in use. As a result, studies evaluating outcomes a week after use may have little value. Finally, her research and that of others have shown that TENS, when applied at adequate intensity and frequency, reduces pain.

Due to lack of evidence, the American College of Physicians makes no recommendation regarding TENS, and the World Health Organization recommends against its use. However, recommendations about the use of TENS are evolving. Low back pain guidelines from the United Kingdom, France, and Austria recommend TENS for some low back pain conditions.

Is it safe?

Overall, TENS is safe. Some people are allergic to the glue that holds the TENS pads in place on the skin (hypoallergenic pads are available for most TENS models), and some find the machine's tingling sensation uncomfortable. TENS should not be used by people with devices implanted in their body, such as cardiac pacemakers or defibrillators, spinal cord stimulators, implanted pump monitors, or any other implanted electronic or metallic devices. Read the manufacturer's instructions for safety.

Is it easily accessible?

TENS units are readily available at some drugstores and pharmacies and online. It is important to look for a unit that allows you to use a mixed-frequency setting, sometimes called SMP mode, so that you can set it to the most effective frequency and intensity. There are numerous options available for between $25 and $100.

Other considerations:

The effectiveness of TENS is still being evaluated. However, it is most likely beneficial when the device is worn over the area of pain and set to a strong but comfortable intensity. Because TENS is safe and relatively inexpensive, it may be worth trying for temporary pain relief, especially while you are engaged in physical activity.

TENS must be applied at the right frequency and intensity to have the best effect. Dr. Sluka's work has shown that using TENS with a mixed-frequency mode—alternating between low and high stimulation frequencies—produces the best effects. She and her research team also found that increasing the intensity to what is sometimes called "strong but comfortable" or "as strong as tolerable" is essential for adequate pain relief. Finally, the electrodes should be placed over the painful area. If you are unclear about how to use your TENS unit based on the directions here, Dr. Sluka and her team have posted free instructions and a video online. Go to the University of Iowa Health Care website and search for TENS. You can also consult your local physical therapist for help with directions.

Bed Rest

Best rest is used to describe refraining from activity as treatment for a medical condition.

How does it work?

The original rationale for bed rest was that limiting body movement would allow the back muscles to heal more quickly. As with lumbar supports and braces, the exact opposite is true. Movement and building core stability are crucial for addressing low back pain.

Is it effective?

Bed rest makes low back pain worse, not better. Guidelines consistently recommend against it.

Is it safe?

Even a short period of bed rest can weaken and destabilize your back muscles over time. In addition, it can make some people more fearful to move and cause them to worry more about what is causing their low back pain. It can also isolate you from family and friends.

Additional Notes

- I have not included a review of dietary supplements in this chapter. There are so many of them that this would require a whole new book. The bottom line is that, except for capsaicin, research does not currently support the use of dietary supplements, and low back pain guidelines do not recommend them.
- I do not address electrical muscle stimulation, laser therapy, or therapeutic ultrasound in this book. Physical therapists and chiropractors sometimes use these passive modalities to treat low back pain, but guidelines do not currently recommend them.
- Keep in mind that the companies that manufacture various treatments for low back pain utilize effective advertising, targeting both

clinicians and people looking for relief. I am suspicious any time I see a treatment advertised as 80 percent effective, because 80 percent of low back pain heals on its own. Be sure to read consumer ratings for low back pain treatments carefully and consider them with a critical eye.

Key Takeaways

- Treatments like ice, superficial heat, and over-the-counter pain medications can provide temporary pain relief but are unlikely to address the underlying Back Factors contributing to low back pain.
- Superficial heat and NSAIDs are recommended by most guidelines for both acute and chronic low back pain, with NSAIDs suggested only after nondrug therapies are tried.
- Cold therapy, lumbar braces, and orthotics are generally not recommended by guidelines due to a lack of clear benefit or limited research.
- Guidelines do not recommend acetaminophen, lidocaine, and menthol topical pain relievers because they do not work better than a placebo and carry some risks.
- For most of these treatments, especially those that are safe and have a low cost, there is little reason not to try them for a short period. However, read customer reviews carefully when choosing a specific manufacturer or device.

chapter 12

Body-Based Treatment Approaches

This chapter focuses on body-based treatment approaches, which include manual therapy techniques and acupuncture. These are some of the most researched treatments for low back pain. Studies consistently show that body-based approaches are safe and have small to moderate effects on low back pain, including pain intensity and physical functioning. As a result, the American College of Physicians calls for patients and clinicians to consider spinal manipulation, massage, and acupuncture before prescription medications. A more recent guideline from the World Health Organization made similar recommendations. Here is why.

Manual Therapy Techniques

Common examples of manual therapy techniques include spinal manipulation, joint mobilization, soft tissue mobilization, and massage. All involve a hands-on approach to moving the joints and/or stimulating the body's soft tissues. As a result, there are many similarities among these techniques. However, there are also distinctions. Some distinctions relate to the technique's overall therapeutic goal, such as spinal manipulation to restore normal joint motion or Swedish massage to reduce muscle spasms. Other distinctions include whether the technique targets joints or soft tissue, and whether it involves a quick thrusting motion or a series of stretching movements. Finally, some distinctions are essentially in name only, based on profession-specific terminology. For instance, a chiropractor might refer to flexion-distraction as spinal manipulation, while an osteopathic physician or a physical therapist might refer to a very similar technique as mobilization.

How does it work?

Similar to exercise, manual therapy techniques can affect multiple body systems, including pain-related processes. The result is increased joint mobility, decreased muscle spasms, less sticky fascia , and changes in the nervous system.

Is it effective?

Among the manual therapy techniques studied, all appear to have similar, mild-to-moderate positive effects on pain and physical functioning. "While many manual therapy technique approaches are different, there isn't a difference in the outcomes," says Chad E. Cook, PT, PhD, director of the Duke Center of Excellence in Manual and Manipulative Therapy and a professor of orthopaedic surgery.

Back Factors:

Manual therapy techniques address multiple Back Factors, including pain associated with arthritis, degenerative joint disease, and muscle spasms. Additionally, there is some evidence that manual therapy techniques can reduce fatigue, improve sleep, decrease stress, and lead to overall improvement in low back pain.

Is it safe?

Manual therapy techniques for the low back are generally safe. The most common side effects are muscle soreness and fatigue, which typically resolve within one to two days. Some people may also experience short-term dizziness, although this is less frequent in manual therapy techniques that focus on the low back. In rare cases, fractures and nerve injuries have occurred. People with underlying conditions such as osteoporosis, inflammatory spine diseases, abdominal aneurysms, infections in the spine, or recent fractures in the spine or pelvis are more likely to experience problems following these treatments. The right healthcare professional will ask you questions about your health history and perform a comprehensive exam on your first visit to see if you have any of these underlying conditions. If so, they will modify their approach to your treatment accordingly.

Healthcare professionals:

Medical physicians may be aware of manual therapies but do not typically offer them. The healthcare professionals most likely to focus on these techniques include chiropractors, physical therapists, and massage therapists. In general, chiropractors focus on spinal manipulation, whereas physical therapists tend to rely more on mobilization techniques. Not surprisingly, massage therapists are most likely to focus on massage. However, training and skill in specific manual therapy techniques are more useful in identifying the right health profession than the initials after their name.

Other considerations:

While manual therapy techniques appear to be similarly effective, this is only true on average. I know from my own experience with low back pain and as a clinician that individual people may respond better to one type of manual therapy than another. What can seem like a miracle cure after one visit for some patients has no effect at all for others. Dr. Cook explains it this way. "Manual therapy techniques impact multiple pain-related systems in our bodies, and they all likely interact with each other in ways that are unique to each person receiving the treatment."

This means it may not always be clear at first which manual therapy will be the most effective for you. Begin by considering what has worked for you in the past, which is most readily available in your community, and what is covered by your health insurance company. Most health insurance, including Medicare and Medicaid, covers at least some manual therapy techniques. However, high co-pays are common, especially if the healthcare professional is out of network. Check with your insurance company in advance to ensure coverage.

Be open to experimenting with different options. Many healthcare professionals specializing in manual therapy offer a range of techniques tailored to the patient's specific needs. This means they can make treatment recommendations tailored to your preferences or symptoms. Having said all this, the more you understand the nuances of each therapy, the easier it is to decide which to start with. To help you make that decision, here is some information on spinal manipulation, joint and soft tissue mobilization, and massage.

Spinal Manipulation

Although other healthcare professionals may perform spinal manipulation, this is the signature treatment of doctors of chiropractic. The three most commonly used (and best researched) techniques are diversified manipulation (also known as high-velocity, low-amplitude [HVLA] or side-posture adjusting), flexion-distraction (also known as low-velocity, variable-amplitude [LVVA] or Cox Technique), and the Activator Method. The main goal of spinal manipulation is to restore normal joint mobility and alleviate pain, but differences in how the techniques are applied matter to some people. Here is a brief description of each.

- **Diversified Manipulation**

  With diversified manipulation to the low back, the patient lies on a narrow table, usually on one side. The clinician ensures the patient is in the proper position, then applies one or more quick thrusts to a specific area of the low back. Depending on the patient's condition, the clinician may apply diversified manipulation to one or both sides of the low back, to the pelvis, or to other areas of the spine.

- **Flexion-Distraction**

  With flexion-distraction, the patient lies face down on a special mechanically assisted table. The clinician gently applies pressure to specific areas of the low back as they move the mechanized table into different positions that flex the hips and, by doing so, distract the spine.

- **The Activator Method**

  The Activator Method uses a small, handheld, spring-loaded device called the Activator Adjusting Instrument. The clinician uses it to apply a rapid low-force thrust into the joints of the spine and pelvis. Unlike the other two techniques I have described, the Activator is used almost exclusively by chiropractors. Because it is a low-force technique, some chiropractors turn to this approach when other types of manipulation are not advised due to osteoporosis, underlying health conditions, or patient preference.

Is it effective?

Most research on spinal manipulation has focused on diversified or flexion-distraction techniques. These studies have found that spinal manipulation leads to a mild-to-moderate decrease in pain and an improvement in physical functioning. More research is needed to compare the effectiveness of specific techniques with one another. In addition to the treatment effects described above for all manual therapy techniques, spinal manipulation may also aid in a process called motor reprogramming. As Robert Vining, DC, DHSc, associate dean of clinical research and professor at Palmer College of Chiropractic, explains it, "When you're in pain, you tend to hold yourself a little differently, move a little differently because you're trying to avoid pain. This different movement puts extra pressure on certain tissues and joints, which also contributes to pain. Spinal manipulation can interrupt the vicious cycle that ensues by improving joint mobility, which in turn helps the muscles and your movements return to a more normal pattern. As a result, the tissues and joints are less likely to be overloaded or irritated. In short, spinal manipulation is intended to help your body return to its pre-pain self."

Low back pain guidelines recommend spinal manipulation for both acute and chronic low back pain. There is also some research, including my own, showing that spinal manipulation may reduce fatigue and improve sleep. Overall, spinal manipulation is safe, as is the case with other manual therapy techniques. Your chiropractor (or other trained healthcare professional) will conduct a history and examination to make sure this treatment is right for you before they recommend spinal manipulation.

People respond differently to spinal manipulation. This is based primarily on the person's underlying condition. For example, some people with acute low back pain will feel better after as few as one or two treatments. People with chronic low back pain or other underlying conditions may take longer to respond. Generally, you should notice a positive response to spinal manipulation after three or four visits. Most people feel better after between six and eight visits. If not, Dr. Vining says, several reasons might explain this:

- Manipulation is not the right treatment for your low back condition.
- Manipulation might work, but you need a different technique.
- The original diagnosis you received was incorrect.
- Manipulation alone is insufficient to address your Back Factors.

If you do not respond to spinal manipulation after a few visits, talk with your healthcare professional about adding other manual therapy techniques or other treatments, such as exercise or mindfulness meditation, to your low back pain care plan. It is also possible that you need a referral to another healthcare professional for further evaluation or a different treatment approach. If you do not find the answers provided by the healthcare professional administering spinal manipulation helpful, consider consulting with another clinician.

Healthcare professionals:

Although chiropractors most commonly offer spinal manipulation, some physical therapists and osteopathic physicians also provide this treatment. See chapter 18 for more information on choosing the right healthcare professional for manual therapy techniques.

Other considerations:

Spinal manipulation can sometimes cause a popping or cracking sound. YouTube is full of examples. While this noise may be startling to some, it is a normal phenomenon. The thrust of the adjustment causes the gas bubbles that form in the fluid surrounding our joints to "pop," resulting in the noise. It does not cause harm to the joint. It also does not indicate whether the adjustment was successful, that is, whether the person will experience less pain or disability following the treatment.

One final note: I mentioned earlier that side-posture adjusting and flexion-distraction are the two most extensively studied spinal manipulation techniques for treating low back pain. If your healthcare professional recommends a different technique, ask them why. The reason should focus on your condition, not the clinician's general preference.

Mobilization

Mobilization is a another hands-on approach to treating low back pain. The clinician slowly and repetitively moves the joints and tissues of the body within their normal range of motion to restore optimal functioning. As Dr. Vining says, "Some people think that mobilization is less forceful than manipulation, but that's not necessarily the case. The difference between manipulation and mobilization does not lie in the force itself. It's repetition and speed."

As is true with manipulation, there are numerous mobilization techniques. Common ones include soft tissue mobilization, joint mobilization, and myofascial release. Soft tissue mobilization involves a combination of stretching and applying deep pressure to the muscles, tendons, and fascia of the low back. It can be very similar to some types of massage. Joint mobilization involves manually moving the joints of the spine slowly through a pain-free range of motion. Myofascial release, also known as "trigger point therapy" targets the fascia. It involves applying steady pressure to painful points in the muscle tissue or gentle stretches to the surrounding soft tissue.

Is it effective?

Although fewer studies have investigated the effects of mobilization, the outcomes are generally similar to manipulation. Guidelines recommend mobilization because it is safe and can decrease pain and improve physical functioning. Mobilization may also help the fluids that flow throughout our bodies, including those that lubricate our joints and fight inflammation, better perform their functions by enhancing circulation in the affected area. The overall effect is ease of movement, which leads to reduced pain and improved physical functioning.

Though it depends on the underlying patient condition, mobilization may be a good place to start for low back pain that is so severe that any movement is really painful. As Dr. Vining explains, "A good clinician will always want to use the intervention that is most tolerated. When someone is in a lot of pain, they may not be able to tolerate much movement, especially quick movements, without exacerbating muscle spasms. Even though spinal manipulation may be otherwise beneficial, if it triggers reflexive bracing that contracts the muscles already in spasm, then you have essentially undone the clinical effect. In these cases, it may be best to start with gentle mobilization procedures."

The recommended number of visits for mobilization is similar to that of spinal manipulation.

Healthcare professionals:

Mobilization is used by physical therapists, many chiropractors, and physicians who practice osteopathic manipulative medicine.

Massage Therapy

Massage therapy involves gentle, controlled pressure on the soft tissues of the body and involves applying rubbing, kneading, or stroking maneuvers over the skin. There are dozens of massage techniques, several of which have been studied for their effect on low back pain and are recommended by guidelines. Examples include Swedish massage, deep tissue massage, trigger point therapy, and sports massage. I have already discussed trigger point therapy above, but here are brief explanations of these other techniques:

- **Swedish Massage**
  The goal of Swedish massage is to create a feeling of relaxation and promote the circulation of blood and other bodily fluids. Movements include circular motions, tapping, vibration, and long, gliding strokes directed toward the soft tissues just under the skin.

- **Deep Tissue Massage**
  Deep tissue massage involves applying slow, firm pressure to the skin to impact the deeper muscles and connective tissue. Trigger point therapy is often part of deep tissue massage. The goal of this technique is to reduce local pain and enhance overall flexibility and body mobility.

- **Sports Massage**
  Sports massage is similar to deep tissue massage. However, deep tissue massage is typically applied to the entire body, while sports massage is more targeted. The healthcare professional tends to focus on specific parts of the body, with an emphasis on areas that are strained or painful due to participation in activities such as sports or shoveling snow.

How does it work?

Massage can help alleviate low back pain by decreasing local inflammation and promoting muscle relaxation. It can also induce a relaxation response that may help address the stress and anxiety commonly associated with low back pain.

Is it effective?

The ACP recommends massage therapy for acute and subacute low back pain, and the WHO recommends it for chronic low back pain. Like other manual therapy techniques, massage is generally considered a safe treatment. You should be able to tell after two or three sessions whether massage will be helpful for your low back pain.

Healthcare professionals:

Chiropractors, physical therapists, and osteopathic physicians may offer brief massage sessions to prepare the patient for spinal manipulation or mobilization. However, massage therapists are most likely to provide full-length massages, typically lasting between thirty and ninety minutes. It is important to work with a massage therapist or other healthcare professional who has experience with individuals who have low back pain.

Other considerations:

People are often completely unclothed or wear only their underwear during a massage. Be sure to talk with your massage therapist if the thought of this makes you feel uncomfortable. Many massage techniques can be applied while the receiver is wholly or partially clothed.

Massage is less likely to be covered by insurance than other manual therapy techniques. Thus, it is best to check with your insurance company about their coverage policies beforehand.

Acupuncture and Dry Needling

Acupuncture involves the insertion of ultrathin needles into specific points in the body along energy channels called meridians. Acupuncture has been a core component of traditional healing practices in China and other East Asian countries for more than 2,500 years. The goal of acupuncture is to improve physiological functioning throughout the entire body. More on this below.

Dry needling is similar to acupuncture in that both use needles. However, this treatment approach was developed independently of acupuncture by American physician Dr. Janet Travell in the 1940s. Rather than placing the needles along meridians, the practitioner places them in trigger points—specific painful areas located in the back muscles. The goal of dry needling is to decrease musculoskeletal pain.

How does it work?

Studies show that acupuncture and dry needling interrupt pain signals that travel from the low back to the brain, release the body's natural painkillers, and help "unwind" sticky or clumped fascia. The result is less low back pain and improved physical functioning. However, there is more to acupuncture than simple pain control. Throughout the centuries, acupuncturists have employed this practice to treat a wide range of diseases and promote overall well-being. The underlying premise is that vital energy, called chi, flows through the body of all living things in channels called meridians. Diseases are believed to be caused by a disruption in the flow of that energy. This disruption can be reversed by inserting acupuncture needles in specific points located along the meridians. If you are interested in delving more deeply into the history and rationale for acupuncture, my favorite book on this topic is *The Web That Has No Weaver* by Ted J. Kaptchuk.

Is it effective?

Studies consistently show that "needling" results in a mild-to-moderate decrease in low back pain intensity and a similar increase in physical functioning. As a result, the ACP recommends acupuncture for acute, subacute, and chronic low back pain, while the WHO recommends it for chronic pain. The number of acupuncture or dry needling treatments required for low back pain will vary depending on the patient's overall health condition. Talk with your provider if you're experiencing any excessive pain or bruising related to needle insertion—they should be able to modify your treatment approach accordingly. Typically, you can expect to feel a positive effect within four to six treatments.

Back Factors:

Acupuncture and dry needling address multiple Back Factors, including pain associated with arthritis, degenerative joint disease, and muscle spasms. Additionally, acupuncture is associated with reduced fatigue, improved sleep, decreased stress, and overall improvement in health and well-being.

Is it safe?

Acupuncture and dry needling are generally considered safe, provided that sterile needles are used and administered by a well-trained healthcare professional. Serious side effects are rare but can include infection at the site where the needle is inserted (this is largely avoided with the use of sterile needles), nerve damage, and, very rarely, lung puncture. Some patients are concerned that acupuncture is painful because it involves needles. However, the needles used are so fine that you often cannot even feel them when they are inserted. Discomfort during needle insertion can include pain or a zinger sensation. Both are usually mild and last for only a moment or two. Tell your acupuncturist right away if the pain lasts longer, as they may want to remove that needle. Temporary mild bleeding can also occur at the insertion site. In rare cases, soreness at the site of needle insertion may last for a day or two, especially with dry needling or in patients with chronic pain conditions.

Healthcare professionals:

Healthcare professionals who offer acupuncture include acupuncturists and doctors of Oriental medicine, as well as some chiropractors and medical physicians who have undergone specialized training. Healthcare professionals who provide dry needling are most likely to be chiropractors, physical therapists, and medical physicians specializing in musculoskeletal pain.

Other considerations:

Acupuncture and dry needling are increasingly available within many healthcare systems nationwide and covered by insurance plans. However, even when acupuncture is covered by insurance, high co-pays are common. As with manual therapy techniques, it is recommended that you call your insurance company in advance to ensure you understand their payment policies.

Key Takeaways

- Manual therapy techniques and acupuncture are among the safest and most effective treatments offered by healthcare professionals for managing low back pain.
- Clinical practice guidelines, such as those from the American College of Physicians and the World Health Organization, recommend manual therapy techniques and acupuncture.
- Common manual therapy techniques for treating low back pain include spinal manipulation, joint and soft tissue mobilization, and massage. These techniques involve hands-on approaches by trained healthcare professionals to manipulate joints and soft tissues, aiming to decrease pain and improve physical functioning.
- Acupuncture involves inserting fine needles into specific points on the body. Practitioners have used this technique for more than 2,500 years to treat various conditions, including low back pain. Dry needling, a Western adaptation, targets specific painful areas called trigger points to alleviate musculoskeletal pain.
- Manual therapy techniques and acupuncture are available in many health systems. These approaches are most likely to be delivered by chiropractors, doctors of osteopathy, physical therapists, massage therapists, and acupuncturists.

chapter 13

Mind-Based Approaches—Mindfulness Meditation

Your thoughts, feelings, and subsequent actions significantly influence how low back pain impacts your daily life. Your mental health affects your physical health, and in turn, your physical health impacts your mental health. Social interactions with others have a profound impact on both. As a result, mind-based treatment approaches that address your thinking, your actions, and the emotional aspects of low back pain can help you lead a more full and active life, even if your pain persists. While mind-based treatments can be beneficial for low back pain in general, guidelines particularly recommend them for individuals with chronic low back pain.

There are many mind-based treatments to choose from and evidence suggests that they are equally effective for low back pain. As a result, you have flexibility in choosing the best approach for you. This chapter focuses on three variations of mindfulness—mindfulness meditation, mindfulness-based stress reduction (MBSR), and progressive muscle relaxation. The next chapter will focus on two psychologically informed treatment approaches: cognitive behavioral therapy and behavioral therapy.

Mindfulness

I briefly touched on mindfulness in chapter 6, and I have used the term a few times already in this chapter. However, for many people, it's not a familiar concept or term. It might even sound a little silly to some of you when I start talking about "being present in the moment." I'll be honest: I was skeptical, too, when I first read those words many years ago. It was only after I reviewed the research and experienced the health benefits of mindfulness firsthand that I realized it is a powerful tool. Powerful enough to be a key component of many of the mind-based treatment options you will learn about next.

What exactly is mindfulness? For the answer to that question, I turned to Duke mindfulness leader and health and wellness coach, Anna Batsakes. Anna describes mindfulness as "the conscious process of slowing the mind down enough to become aware of what is happening both around and within you, right here, right now, in this moment, without judgment."

One way to cultivate mindfulness is to become more aware of what is happening in your body. This is sometimes called body awareness. When you focus on your breathing, whether your muscles are tense or loose, or if you are hungry or tired, you automatically ground yourself in the present moment. Tuning in to your body keeps you more attuned to your needs—whether it's taking a deep breath, adjusting your posture, eating when you are hungry, or resting when you are tired. As a result, mindfulness enhances body awareness, while body awareness deepens mindfulness.

Mindfulness and Body Awareness Exercise

Paying attention to yourself (your changing thoughts, sensations, and emotions) and the world around you allows you to become more aware of the connection between your mind and your body. Greater awareness of that connection can help you master your low back pain.

1. Sit quietly and take a couple of deep breaths.
2. Then ask yourself the question "What is going on inside my body right now?"
3. Tune inward as you notice your breath, any pain you might be experiencing, or areas where you are relaxed versus those where you are holding stress. Tight shoulders, a clenched jaw, or stiff back muscles might indicate areas of stress.

Sitting quietly in this way for three to five minutes is one way to be mindful, but almost anything can be turned into a mindfulness exercise. Here are some options. Try paying total attention to the feel and taste of food the next time you eat, or fully focusing on the sound of the birds (or the wind through the trees) during your next walk. Paying attention to yourself (your changing thoughts, sensations, and emotions) and the world around you allows you to become more aware of the connection between your mind and your body. Greater awareness of that connection can help you master your low back pain.

Mindfulness Meditation

"All meditation is mindfulness, but not all mindfulness is meditation," says Anna. The mindfulness part of mindfulness meditation involves noticing what is happening in one's inner and outer environment. The meditation part is a state in which the mind becomes freer, able to let go of "thought clutter" and any judgment about one's thoughts or life circumstances. Mindfulness meditation practices are increasingly being adopted by healthcare professionals as the evidence of their effectiveness in treating a broad range of health conditions grows. However, mindfulness meditation has existed as part of Hindu and Buddhist healing traditions for thousands of years.

How does it work?

Researchers are still learning the answer to this question. Here is some of what is known so far. Chronic pain can change the areas of the brain that process pain, causing us to experience more pain and lessening our ability to tolerate it as time goes on. Mind-focused therapies may "reroute" the brain in the opposite direction. As a result, pain decreases, and the remaining pain becomes less bothersome. Mindfulness meditation is also thought to reduce pain by interrupting nerve pathways that carry pain signals to and from the brain.

Is it effective?

Studies suggest mindfulness meditation can decrease pain levels and improve physical functioning in people with chronic low back pain. This practice can also improve sleep quality and overall well-being, including helping individuals better manage their pain. Mindfulness meditation combined with cognitive behavioral therapy may also help people become less reliant on pain medications, including opioids.

Back Factors:

Mindfulness meditation directly addresses several Back Factors, including stress, anxiety, depression, fear avoidance, ONTs, sleep quality, and fatigue. It can also help with overall health and well-being.

Is it safe?

Mindfulness meditation is safe. One caveat. Don't engage in mindfulness meditation while performing activities that require your full attention, such as driving. Also, some people experience mental distress and anxiety while trying to meditate. If this happens to you, consider talking with a pain psychologist or mindfulness coach about ways to address these feelings or emotions.

Is it easily accessible?

There are many ways to turn one's attention inward and maintain focus there for a specified period of time. Paying attention to your breath is one way to stay grounded and in the present moment. Some people focus on the soft glow of a lit candle instead. Others pick a sentence or phrase with meaning to them (a mantra) and silently repeat it over and over. Another option is to use an app or join a class that guides you through the meditation process. Prayer can also be a form of meditation. Experiment to learn which approach or approaches works best for you. It is normal for the mind to get distracted by thoughts during meditation. When this happens, notice those thoughts, let them flow by like clouds, and return the mind's focus to the breath, the candle, or the mantra.

This is all easier said than done for most of us. Fortunately, numerous resources are available to help you get started with mindfulness meditation. Examples include books such as *Meditations for Mortals*, by Oliver Burkeman, and *Think Like a Monk*, by Jay Shetty, as well as apps like Calm, Headspace, and Insight Timer. Many health systems, including those at Duke, Harvard, and Stanford, offer mindfulness resources and training.

In the meantime, following is a mindfulness meditation exercise you can try now.

Mindfulness Meditation Exercise

1. **Decide how long you wish to meditate and set a timer.**

   Start small. Five minutes can seem like a long time when you first get started!

2. **Sit quietly for a moment.**

   Close your eyes, or if that feels uncomfortable, soften your gaze as you look forward.

3. **Take a deep breath in and then exhale slowly.**

   Do this a couple of times.

4. **Start paying attention to the things happening around you.**

   Maybe you hear the sound of traffic, or music playing in the background, or the murmur of voices in the next room. Notice the feel of the air against your skin or your feet on the floor. Don't dwell on any particular thing. Notice it and then let it go. Focus instead on your breath as you slowly inhale through your nose and exhale through your mouth.

5. **Expect your mind to get distracted by your thoughts.**

   One goal of meditation is to give your minds a break from your thoughts. Even tiny breaks allow the thinker to gain a better perspective on current thought patterns and gently shift those patterns into more positive, supportive ways of thinking.

6. **Interrupt your thought patterns by asking yourself, "I wonder what I will think of next," and then wait to find out.**

   - Let that thought float in and then out of your mind, simply noticing.
   - Then, make a conscious decision about what to think next. Pick something familiar, such as picturing your favorite place (e.g., reclining on a beach or by a lake), and recall how much you enjoy it.
   - When you feel ready, let go of the thought.
   - Repeat by asking yourself once again, "I wonder what I will think of next." Expect to be distracted repeatedly. When that distraction happens, notice those thoughts, too. Let them flow by like a cloud in the sky or a fish in the ocean. Practice non-judgment as you do so.

7. **Return your focus to your breath.**

8. **Continue this process until the timer expires.**

   When it does, take a couple more deep breaths.

9. **Open your eyes if they are closed and bring yourself back to the present moment.**

Mindfulness-Based Stress Reduction

Mindfulness-based stress reduction (MBSR) was developed in the 1970s by Dr. Jon Kabat-Zinn, bestselling author and professor at the University of Massachusetts Medical School. This approach is recommended by many healthcare professionals for patients living with a range of diseases and conditions, including chronic low back pain.

MBSR includes mindfulness meditation as part of a more comprehensive stress management program. MBSR requires a significantly larger time commitment than the other mind-based approaches described in this chapter and is likely to be most helpful for people with chronic pain. It involves eight structured group sessions (one per week) led by one or more instructors. In addition to mindfulness meditation, MBSR also includes yoga and group discussions. Yoga adds an exercise component. Group discussions, focused on stress management and individual group members' experiences with practicing mindfulness, can help foster a sense of community and address the isolation that people with long-standing chronic low back pain often experience. Research shows that MBSR and other mind-based approaches are equally effective. Programs are available both in person and virtually at major academic institutions across the United States. You can also learn more about MBSR by reading one of Dr. Kabat-Zinn's books, such as *Mindfulness for Beginners* or *Full Catastrophe Living*.

Progressive Muscle Relaxation

Progressive muscle relaxation was developed by Dr. Edmund Jacobson more than one hundred years ago. This mind-based approach is closely related to mindfulness meditation but is more body focused. It involves methodically tensing and then releasing the main muscle groups in your body one at a time while simultaneously paying attention to the sensations that occur in the muscles. The goal is to reduce stress and muscle tension, leading to a state of complete relaxation. Because it directly targets the muscles of the body, progressive muscle relaxation may be particularly beneficial in relieving low back muscle spasms. If you do it before bedtime, it may help you fall asleep more easily. Progressive muscle relaxation is the mind-based technique that I use most often, usually right before going to sleep at night.

If you'd like to try this for yourself, here is the exercise I use.

Progressive Muscle Relaxation Exercise

1. **Lie flat on your back with your hands at your sides.**

2. **Take a couple of deep breaths.**

3. **Contract your muscles throughout your body.**

    - Direct your attention to your right leg. As you breathe in, draw your leg muscles inward toward your leg bones, squeezing tightly all the way up from your toes to your thighs. Hold for a few seconds. Exhale and release the squeeze. Repeat with the left leg.

    - Next, squeeze and release the muscles in your buttocks.

    - Then, move to your spine. Starting at the very bottom of your spine, squeeze the muscles in your lower back and release. Move to your middle back, squeeze, and release. Do the same with your upper back, and then your neck.

    - Next, squeeze and release your abdominal muscles, followed by your middle and upper chest.

- Then move to the muscles in your right arm, squeezing in from your fingers to your shoulders. Repeat with your left arm.
- Squeeze your shoulders up toward your ears.
  Hold and release.
- Now scrunch up all the muscles in your face.
  Hold and release.

4. **Relax your muscles throughout your body.**
   - Starting at the tips of your toes, slowly take a deep breath in as you more deeply relax the muscles of your feet, ankles, calves, thighs, and buttocks. Exhale.
   - Take another breath and repeat the exercise with your arms, starting with your fingers and working your way up to your shoulders.
   - Next is your spine. Slowly relax the muscles of your back, starting at the base of your spine and working your way up to the top of your head.
   - Then move on to relaxing the muscles of your face, softening your jaw, slightly parting your lips, letting your eyes sink back into your skull.
5. **Take a few more deep breaths and feel yourself sink deeper into the floor or bed with each breath that you take.**
6. **Remain in this position, focusing on your breath, as long as you like.**

Key Takeaways

- Mind-based therapies like mindfulness meditation are especially effective for managing chronic low back pain.
- Mindfulness improves body awareness and emotional regulation by helping you stay present and attuned to your physical and mental state.
- Mindfulness meditation can reduce pain by altering brain pathways and improving sleep, mood, and medication reliance.
- Mindfulness-based stress reduction combines meditation, yoga, and group support to address chronic pain holistically.
- Progressive muscle relaxation relieves physical tension and stress by systematically tensing and relaxing muscle groups.

chapter 14

Mind-Based Approaches—Psychological Treatments

This chapter continues the discussion of mind-based treatment options by describing cognitive behavioral therapy (CBT) and behavioral therapy. Before I dive into the specifics of these mind-based therapies, there is an issue that I want to hit head on. Several of the healthcare professionals I interviewed for this book brought up the issue of bias and stigma associated with depression, anxiety, fear avoidance, ONTs, and other mental health conditions. Many inroads have been made over the last decade or so when it comes to supporting people experiencing mental health conditions. However, some people remain dismissive of health conditions that cannot be seen or measured by objective tests. Remember the "all in your head" discussion from chapter 3? That dismissive stance is even more common when low back pain is associated with mental health challenges. As a result, psychological treatment approaches can be met with skepticism by both patients and some healthcare professionals. If this is true for you, pain psychologist Dr. Robert Kerns recommends you acknowledge those feelings up front. Then work to replace those old beliefs with new information. Also, keep in mind that the psychologically-based approaches currently used to treat chronic low back pain are very different from the insight or talk psychotherapies that might be most familiar to you. Instead, psychological treatments for low back pain tend to be short-term structured sessions that are primarily educational in nature.

Psychological therapies can be effective even when people are initially very skeptical. Dr. Kerns says that the right mental health professional will respect your beliefs and address your skepticism early on in a way that can help you become engaged. Prior beliefs matter, but they aren't necessarily the barrier to successful treatment that some might think. "Psychological treatment can result in a reduction in pain intensity, improved physical functioning, social role functioning, and overall quality of life," says Dr. Kerns. "So, it's worth your investment to give these approaches a try."

Cognitive Behavioral Therapy

The mind-based practices you explored in the last chapter focused on calming the mind and body. Cognitive behavioral therapy (CBT) relies on some of the same techniques, but its principles differ. The primary goal of CBT is to change the thoughts and behaviors that work against our ability to deal with pain. Rather than buying into overly negative thoughts and being resigned to negative beliefs about one's pain, CBT practices encourage people to challenge harmful thoughts and beliefs, develop a sense of calm, and foster new and healthier thinking, feeling, and behavior patterns.

CBT encourages behavior change using specific strategies. One strategy is activity pacing, which involves two steps. The first step is to listen to the body and determine when to be active and when to rest. The second step is to gradually increase activity over time by alternating periods of moderate activity with limited rest breaks. Remember Chris from chapter 7? He described how, on some days, he can clean his whole house. On other days, it is best to focus on smaller tasks instead. This is an excellent example of pacing. Another strategy is to become more physically active. People with low back pain are often fearful about movement and, as a result, limit their daily activities. Think about how exercise helped Robert, Valerie, and Joel lessen their low back pain and lead more active lives. Behavioral activation is a third CBT strategy. Behavioral activation involves systematically engaging in meaningful activities that are being avoided out of fear. The goal is to discover which activities can still be enjoyed, even if some pain is envolved.

How does it work?

> ***Dr. Francis Keefe explains how CBT works:***
>
> *As low back pain becomes chronic, it changes how the brain functions. As a result, one begins to pay more attention to their pain, and it becomes more challenging to deal with. For some people, it may become difficult to think*

about anything else. Fear follows. They worry about what might be causing the pain or how pain and disability will impact the future. These repetitive thoughts lead to further brain changes, increasing pain sensitivity. The pain gets worse as a result. To add fuel to this vicious cycle, a large percentage of people with low back pain also experience stress, anxiety, or depression. These emotions can further intensify the perception of pain. Fear may lead a person to avoid physical and social activities. The result is less movement and increased social isolation, both of which also exacerbate low back pain. CBT helps to break this vicious cycle by teaching people how to navigate the emotional aspects of pain. This in turn increases their levels of social and physical activity, which in turn decreases their thoughts about pain, which in turn reduces the amount of pain they experience.

Diane Solomon, PhD, an adjunct professor at Oregon Health and Science University and a writer for *Psychology Today*, agrees with Dr. Keefe about the vicious cycle. Here she describes how to overcome it.

Dr. Solomon explains:

You feel a twinge in your low back. Automatically, your first thoughts are, "I just felt a twinge. My low back pain is going to get worse. I am going to end up in the hospital, just like I did last time." And you're off to the (painful) races. CBT teaches us to think differently, to interrupt and change that maladaptive thought pattern. Instead of catastrophizing (ONTs), you can think, "I just felt a twinge. It could get worse, but it could also get better. I have new behavioral skills to utilize, such as stretching or breathing exercises, and my new cognitive skills to challenge the automatic thought that things will get worse. I have dealt with this before and can do it again. I have people to call for help or support. I've got this."

With meditation, you observe your thoughts and then release them. With CBT, you challenge those mindful thoughts by using cognitive skills. An example is developing more helpful thought alternatives, such as "I know it is difficult, but I have several strategies and can handle this pain." You can also use a technique called thought stopping. If you catch yourself going down a thought-clutter spiral, tell yourself to stop. Imagine a stop sign. Once you stop an overly negative thought, the next step is to implement behavioral skills, such as stretching, going for a walk, or creating alternative scenarios. The result is twofold. Not only will you have less low back pain now, but because you are changing the neural pathways in your brain, you are also less likely to experience debilitating low back pain in the future.

See Tables 14.1 and 14.2 for examples of how alternative scenarios work. The percentages (%) in the tables refer to the level of certainty a person might have that specific scenarios will happen. For example, if you are certain you will end up in the hospital because of your low back pain, rate it at 100%. If you think it is very unlikely to happen but still possible, rate it at 10% or 20%. Many people start out estimating the likelihood of various scenarios in a way that is similar to those outlined in Table 14.1. As you see, the bad outcomes (mind clutter) are rated as more likely than the more positive alternative scenarios.

Table 14.1: Starting Scenarios

Scenario	% chance this is true
I felt a twinge in my lower back.	100%
Mind Clutter	**% chance this is true**
I am going to end up in the hospital again.	95%
My life is ruined forever.	80%
Alternative Scenarios	**% chance this is true**
I can take a couple of deep breaths and do some stretching exercises. The last time I did that, the pain went away.	10%

Alternative Scenarios cont.	% chance this is true
I can also take two Advil and a hot bath. That has also worked in the past.	30%
If my pain is still there in the morning, I will make an appointment with my physical therapist or chiropractor. That always helps.	15%
I will probably be fine in a day or two.	5%

However, with effort and time, many people find that their estimates on the likelihood of these different scenarios begin to shift in a more positive direction. See Table 14.2 for how this might look.

Table 14.2: Scenarios after 30 Days of CBT Training

Scenario	% chance this is true
I felt a twinge in my lower back.	100%
Mind Clutter	**% chance this is true**
I am going to end up in the hospital again.	20%
My life is ruined forever.	15%
Alternative Scenarios	**% chance this is true**
I can take a couple of deep breaths and do some stretching exercises. The last time I did that, the pain went away.	80%
I can also take two Advil and a hot bath. That has also worked in the past.	90%

Alternative Scenarios cont.	% chance this is true
If my pain is still there in the morning, I will make an appointment with my physical therapist or chiropractor. That always helps.	70%
I will probably be fine in a day or two.	55%

Dr. Solomon says it is okay if you really believe the negative mind clutter and honestly think the alternative scenarios are hogwash. Research shows that this doesn't matter: If you continue practicing CBT, your percentages will shift and you'll start to see the results.

Is it effective?

Research shows that CBT can lead to reduced pain, improved function, and less emotional distress. As a result, it is commonly recommended by guidelines for the treatment of low back pain, especially when it is chronic.

Back Factors:

Similar to mindfulness meditation, CBT directly addresses the following Back Factors: stress, anxiety, depression, fear avoidance, ONTs, sleep quality, and fatigue.

Is it safe?

CBT is generally considered to be a safe treatment approach for addressing low back pain. However, some people may temporarily feel uncomfortable, stressed, or anxious during and after CBT sessions. This therapeutic approach requires individuals to face challenging thoughts and feelings that are contributing to their low back pain. A skilled mental health professional can help you deal with these thoughts and feelings if they occur.

Is it easily accessible?

Many mental health professionals, including psychologists and social workers who specialize in pain management, receive training on how to use CBT safely and effectively. Unfortunately, "available" does not always translate into "accessible." There is a limited number of mental health providers with specific training, background, interests, expertise, and competencies around the delivery of evidence-based psychological treatments for pain. As a result, health systems frequently have months-long wait times for appointments with a pain psychologist or social worker.

Here are a few alternatives:

1. **Consider seeking a healthcare professional in your area or online who is trained in the Empowered Relief program.** Pain psychologist and Stanford University professor of anesthesiology, perioperative and pain medicine Beth Darnall, PhD, developed Empowered Relief. Her goal was to address the access problem I just described. She created Empowered Relief, a two-hour intervention that rapidly equips patients with pain relief skills, including those in CBT, mindfulness, and pain neuroscience education. A recent research study evaluating Empowered Relief for patients with low back pain found that those who completed Empowered Relief experienced reductions in pain intensity, pain interference, pain-related distress, sleep disturbance, anxiety, and depression that were similar to what patients experienced after an eight-session CBT program. As I write this book, more than two thousand healthcare professionals around the world have been certified to provide the Empowered Relief program, including some who work at the Cleveland Clinic and the VHA. You can search the Empowered Relief website under Find a Provider to learn if one of these healthcare professionals is located near you, or you can search for a certified instructor who offers online classes to registrants from all areas.

2. **Expand the reach of your search parameters.**

   The growing use of telehealth sometimes makes it possible to schedule a virtual visit with a licensed psychologist who is located in the state where you live but whose office is too far away for in-person visits.

3. **Look for evidence-based psychological approaches you can do on your own.**

   Consider books or technology-driven approaches. One example is Dr. Rachel Zoffness's *The Pain Management Workbook,* available online and in many bookstores. Another example is a free eight-week online CBT program codeveloped by Dr. Keefe, which you can find by searching the internet for paintrainer.org.

Behavioral Therapy

The goal of behavioral therapy is to increase active involvement in daily activities and decrease the tendency to engage in pain-related behaviors that can work against you (e.g., spending too much time in the recliner). As Dr. Solomon describes it, "You do something to help you, and you avoid doing something that isn't helping you." Patients are encouraged to reward themselves when they (1) avoid behaviors that exacerbate low back pain, such as bed rest, inactivity, and overuse of pain medications, or (2) engage in daily activities that are helpful, such as exercise and meditation. The rewards can be simple, such as going out for coffee with a friend or listening to one's favorite music while going on a walk. Some activities are intrinsically rewarding, for instance, seeing a movie that you really enjoy with your best friend. Others are more extrinsic, for example, focusing on behaviors that promote activity and function in the long run, such as exercising even when you don't really feel like it.

How does it work?

The goal of behavioral therapy is to improve overall physical functioning by gradually increasing a person's activity levels, reducing fear avoidance behaviors, and breaking the cycle of disability and pain that Dr. Keefe described earlier.

Is it effective?

Research shows that behavioral therapy is effective in treating chronic low back pain, especially for those who are disabled or rely heavily on pain medications. The World Health Organization recommends this treatment approach for chronic low back pain.

Back Factors:

Behavioral therapy is beneficial for patients experiencing fear avoidance and ONTs.

Is it safe?

The safety of behavioral therapy is similar to that of CBT. Work with a trained and experienced mental health professional if you choose to try this treatment approach for low back pain.

Is it easily accessible?

Access to behavioral therapy is similar to that of CBT.

Other considerations:

Behavioral therapy works best when combined with other treatments, like exercise or CBT. Not surprisingly, this approach is most effective for individuals who are highly motivated to change their pain-related behaviors and who live in a supportive environment.

A Final Note

Pain psychologist Dr. Kerns has had many people experiencing chronic low back pain with mental health conditions tell him that their lives would be fine if it were not for the pain. "If you had my pain, you'd be depressed, too," or "You need to fix my pain, and then I won't be depressed." Unfortunately, having the pain go away is not necessarily the complete answer for some people. While a course of CBT may help with low back pain, there is very little evidence that it will help with serious mental health conditions. If you believe you might have a major depressive disorder, substance abuse, or generalized anxiety disorder, it is important to seek care from a healthcare professional who focuses on these conditions.

Key Takeaways

- Cognitive behavioral therapy (CBT) and behavioral therapy are structured, evidence-based psychological treatments that help manage chronic low back pain by addressing harmful thought patterns and promoting healthier behaviors.
- Research shows that CBT can significantly reduce pain intensity, improve functioning, and enhance quality of life.
- CBT breaks the vicious cycle of chronic pain by teaching individuals to challenge negative thoughts, engage in meaningful activities, and rewire brain pathways associated with pain perception.

- Behavioral therapy focuses on reinforcing positive daily actions and discouraging pain-related behaviors, using rewards to motivate increased activity and social engagement.
- Access to trained professionals for these therapies can be limited, but telehealth, self-guided programs like paintrainer.org, and short-format options like Stanford's Empowered Relief offer promising alternatives.

chapter 15

Prescription Medications

The decision whether or not to take prescription medications for your low back pain is one that only you can make, in partnership with your medical physician, nurse practitioner, or physician assistant. Because this is a partnership, it is important that you be as informed as possible on the general risks and benefits of prescriptions before you walk into your healthcare professional's office. The purpose of this chapter is to help you with this task by providing a brief overview of the medications most commonly used for low back pain. You will find information on how these drugs work, how well they work, and their potential side effects. Along the way, you will meet three primary care physicians who share their opinions based on decades of research and experience in treating patients with low back pain who are taking prescription medications.

Why are decisions about the use of medication so complicated? There are several reasons. First, the use of medication for low back pain is widespread. Prescription medication as the answer to whatever ails us is a core part of our biomedical culture. Second, at least half of people with low back pain who see a health professional start out with their primary care physician, and prescriptions are a common tool in their toolbox. Third, low back pain usually heals on its own. If that healing occurs after taking a pill, the person taking it may assume the pill worked even when it had little or no real effect. In chapter 7, I explained how powerful the mind can be. It turns out that the mind is so powerful that healing can sometimes occur even when the treatment itself has no real healing ability. This phenomenon, called the placebo effect, is well recognized by researchers and clinicians. Scientists use it as a research tool, comparing new medications to a placebo (a sugar pill) to determine whether the medications are safe and effective.

The reason for taking medication is not that it cures low back pain. Pills do not address the underlying causes of low back pain or any Back Factors. It is not because prescription medications are universally effective. In most cases, pills either work just a little or don't work at all for low back pain. It is not because prescription medications are safe. All pills carry some risk of harm, ranging from only risky for some people to very risky for pretty much everyone. It is not because low back pain guidelines widely recommend prescription medications. Recall that the ACP recommends nondrug treatment approaches for low back pain before any prescription medications are tried. The WHO is even less enthusiastic about medication, recommending only NSAIDs and topical cayenne pepper. In addition, the WHO specifically recommends against taking skeletal muscle relaxants, glucocorticoids (such as prednisone), antidepressant medications, and opioids.

As Jon Lurie, MD, MS, professor of medicine and orthopaedics in the Geisel School of Medicine at Dartmouth, explains it, "Prescription pain medication may be a good option for people who have tried pretty much every nondrug approach, and nothing has worked. They are still living with a level of pain that makes it difficult for them to function. That is when it is worth trying medication—to see if it takes the edge off their pain so that they can remain active and maintain some quality of life."

Now, on to specific prescriptions commonly used for low back pain. Skeletal muscle relaxants, duloxetine, and tramadol are listed first because they are recommended by the American College of Physicians' low back pain guideline if nondrug therapies are not effective. The other medications listed are commonly used for low back pain but either are not recommended or guidelines recommend against their use.

One final note before getting started. I already covered NSAIDs and acetaminophen in the last chapter since they are available over the counter. I won't mention them again here, but keep in mind that both these medications are available at higher doses with a prescription. The same benefits and risks apply, but those risks increase with higher doses.

Skeletal Muscle Relaxants

As the name implies, skeletal muscle relaxants are primarily used to relax muscle spasms and spasticity. They are available as pills. Common examples of those used for low back pain include cyclobenzaprine (Flexeril) and carisoprodol (Soma).

How does it work?

Skeletal muscle relaxants work by slowing down the transmission of pain signals traveling in the nerves between the spinal cord and the brain.

Is it effective?

Additional research is needed to more definitively answer questions about the effectiveness of skeletal muscle relaxants for low back pain. The available studies are mostly of low quality and, as a result, are less trustworthy sources of evidence. Some studies have found that skeletal muscle relaxants are no more helpful than a placebo in treating low back pain, while others have found a small positive effect for acute low back pain. That effect is probably not enough to make a difference to most people. Despite the lack of strong evidence, physicians commonly prescribe skeletal muscle relaxants. The ACP recommends their use for acute low back pain if non-drug treatments are not helpful. The WHO guideline recommends against the use of skeletal muscle relaxants for the treatment of chronic low back pain.

Is it safe?

Although the effectiveness of skeletal muscle relaxants is debated, the risks are clear. Side effects may include nausea, blurred vision, headache, fatigue, sleepiness, dizziness, and potential interactions with other medications, especially medications that affect the nervous system. There is also a rare but real possibility of liver damage.

Is it easily accessible?

Any medical physician can prescribe skeletal muscle relaxants. In most states, they can also be prescribed by nurse practitioners and physician assistants.

Other considerations:

The side effects of skeletal muscle relaxants may be more dangerous for older adults due to an increased risk of falls.

Duloxetine

Duloxetine, often known by the brand name Cymbalta, is a serotonin-norepinephrine reuptake inhibitor taken as a pill.

How does it work?

Duloxetine increases the amount of two naturally occurring chemicals found in the brain—serotonin and norepinephrine. The job of these chemicals is to regulate your moods and your perception of pain.

Is it effective?

Duloxetine may reduce low back pain and improve physical functioning. The ACP recommends this medication as a second-line treatment if guideline-recommended nondrug treatments and NSAIDs are not effective. However, the WHO recommends against the use of serotonin-norepinephrine reuptake inhibitors as the benefits may not outweigh the risks for many people.

Is it safe?

Side effects include stomach and intestinal problems, sleepiness, dizziness, headaches, sexual dysfunction, muscle pain and cramps, tingling sensations, weight changes, and sweating. More serious risks include addiction, severe liver damage, sudden drops in blood pressure, problems with urination, suicidal thoughts (especially in teenagers), bleeding, glaucoma, seizures, and a condition called serotonin syndrome.

Serotonin syndrome is a potentially fatal condition caused when the level of serotonin (a chemical in your brain that regulates sleep and mood) gets too high.

Is it easily accessible?

Any medical physician can prescribe duloxetine. In most states, this medication can also be prescribed by nurse practitioners and physician assistants.

Tramadol

Tramadol is an opioid that has some similarities to duloxetine. Tramadol is available as a pill under the brand names Ultram, Ultram ER, Conzip, and Qdolo.

How does it work?

Tramadol acts in the body in two ways. First, this drug binds to opioid receptor sites in the brain, meaning the way it affects the body is similar to the way other opioids affect the body. Second, tramadol increases serotonin and norepinephrine levels in the brain, similar to duloxetine.

Is it effective?

Tramadol may decrease low back pain, but it is unclear if it works better than NSAIDs, and the risk of side effects is significantly greater. Although the ACP recommends tramadol if other approaches are ineffective, the WHO recommends against it, as the benefits do not outweigh the risks for most people.

Is it safe?

The side effects of tramadol are similar to those of both opioids and duloxetine, including the risk of abuse/addiction. This drug can also cause irregular heart rhythms and, in some cases, make low back pain worse.

Is it easily accessible?

Any medical physician can prescribe tramadol. In some states, this drug can also be prescribed by nurse practitioners and physician assistants.

Oral Steroids

Oral steroids such as prednisone (Deltasone), methylprednisolone (Medrol), and dexamethasone (Maxidex, Ozurdex, and Dexpak) are available as pills. They are powerful anti-inflammatory medications sometimes prescribed for acute low back pain, especially when sciatica is present.

How does it work?

Steroids are potent anti-inflammatory drugs used to target inflammation occurring in the spinal nerves, nerve roots, or intervertebral discs. They work by mimicking cortisol, a naturally occurring hormone, to suppress inflammation. However, steroids also suppress the ability to fight off infections.

Is it effective?

Oral steroids may slightly decrease pain and improve physical functioning, but only for a very short period and only when radicular pain is present. Because their impact on pain is not significant and the side effects can be serious, oral steroids are not recommended by low back pain guidelines. In particular, the WHO recommends against their use.

Is it safe?

Oral steroids are associated with a whole host of short-term side effects, including high blood pressure, increased blood sugar, weight gain, swelling, trouble sleeping, anxiety, irritability, nausea, and heartburn. In the long run, oral steroids can cause problems with the ability to fight infections, an increased risk of bone fractures, glaucoma, cataracts, and a disease called Cushing's syndrome.

Is it easily accessible?

Any medical physician can prescribe oral steroids. In most states, they can also be prescribed by nurse practitioners and physician assistants.

Other considerations:

The active ingredient in both oral steroids and corticosteroid injections (see chapter 16, on interventional procedures) is the same steroid medication. However, oral steroids enter the bloodstream and move throughout the entire body. With injections, the medication stays local to the low back. In most cases, oral steroids are prescribed for short periods (less than a week), often for acute low back pain.

Gabapentin

Gabapentin, also called Neurontin, Gralise, or Horizant, comes as a pill. For the low back, it is most often used to treat neuropathic pain, including sciatica.

How does it work?

Gabapentin slows the transmission of nerve signals between the spinal cord and the brain.

Is it effective?

Gabapentin is not effective in the treatment of low back pain. It does not reduce pain or improve physical functioning. As a result, it is not approved by the Food and Drug Administration for low back pain or recommended by low back pain guidelines. The WHO specifically recommends against its use.

Is it safe?

Common side effects include sleepiness, dizziness, headaches, nausea and vomiting, weight gain, and swelling in the arms and legs. Gabapentin can also cause breathing problems, lead to severe allergic reactions, addiction, and sexual dysfunction, damage the kidneys and liver, and cause anxiety, depression, and suicidal thoughts. Gabapentin should not be taken with other drugs, including antidepressants, alcohol, and opioids. Some studies also suggest a link between gabapentin and dementia.

Is it easily accessible?

Any medical physician can prescribe gabapentin. In most states, this drug can also be prescribed by nurse practitioners and physician assistants.

Other considerations:

Gabapentin may be worth the risks in treating some diseases, including shingles and seizures caused by epilepsy. However, this medication should be avoided when it comes to low back pain.

Pregabalin

Pregabalin is available as a pill under the brand name Lyrica. Pregabalin is most often used to treat seizures and fibromyalgia but is sometimes also used for neuropathic low back pain, including sciatica. Pregabalin is related to gabapentin in that both are classified as gabapentinoids, but they are not the same drug. Pregabalin is a more potent medication than gabapentin and begins to work more quickly.

How does it work?

Pregabalin slows the transmission of nerve signals between the spinal cord and the brain.

Is it effective?

Similar to gabapentin, pregabalin is not effective in treating low back pain when compared to a placebo and is associated with substantial side effects. The WHO specifically recommends against its use for low back pain.

Is it safe?

The side effects of pregabalin are similar to those of gabapentin.

Is it easily accessible?

Any medical physician can prescribe pregabalin, but it is considered a controlled substance, so there are extra steps involved in the process. In some states, it can also be prescribed by nurse practitioners and physician assistants.

Other considerations:

Pregabalin is more likely to lead to misuse, abuse, and addiction than many other pain medications, including gabapentin.

Benzodiazepines

Benzodiazepines are drugs taken in pill form. This drug is sold under several brand names, including Xanax, Klonopin, Valium, Ativan, and Halcion.

How does it work?

Benzodiazepines slow down nerve activity by increasing the effects of GABA, one of the brain's neurotransmitters. This slowed-down effect leads people to feel calmer and less anxious.

Is it effective?

Benzodiazepines are not effective in treating low back pain when compared to either placebo (sugar pills) or other treatment approaches. Guidelines for low back pain are either silent on the use of benzodiazepines or, as is the case with the WHO, specifically recommend against their use.

Is it safe?

Sleepiness and dizziness are common side effects. The biggest safety issue with benzodiazepines is that people can become addicted. They can also lead to potentially fatal overdoses, especially when taken in combination with opioids or alcohol. When used for long periods, benzodiazepines can also interfere with the ability to think clearly and recall past events.

Is it easily accessible?

Any medical physician can prescribe benzodiazepines, but they are considered a controlled substance, so there are extra steps involved in the process. In some states, they can also be prescribed by nurse practitioners and physician assistants.

Other considerations:

While benzodiazepines are primarily used to treat anxiety and panic disorder, some physicians feel that they may have a muscle-relaxing effect and also prescribe them to treat low back pain.

Opioids

There are several different types of opioids, including morphine, codeine, oxycodone, hydrocodone, methadone, and fentanyl. Some opioids, such as morphine and codeine, are natural products derived from the poppy plant. Others, like methadone and fentanyl, are manufactured chemical compounds based on naturally occurring opioids. Opioids are available in pill form, as a patch or a nasal spray, or via an infusion. Common brand names include OxyContin and Vicodin.

How does it work?

Opioids act at receptor sites that control pain and mood. As a result, people who take them may experience less pain, less worry about pain, or a feeling of euphoria or being "high."

Is it effective?

Opioids do not work any better for low back pain than other medications, such as NSAIDs, or much better than a placebo. The Centers for Disease Control and Prevention (CDC), the ACP, and the WHO all recommend against the use of opioids whenever possible because there are other drugs and nonpharmacological treatments (e.g., spinal manipulation and exercise) that are as effective and associated with much less risk of harm.

Is it safe?

Side effects include constipation, sleepiness, feeling "high," nausea, and vomiting. There is also a significant risk of increased tolerance, addiction, overdose, and death. According to the CDC, more than three hundred thousand Americans died from prescription opioid overdoses between 1999 and 2023. When you include deaths from illegal opioids like heroin and illicit fentanyl, the total number of opioid-related deaths rises to over eight hundred thousand. Despite growing awareness of the risks, opioid use still remains too widespread. According to the CDC, medical physicians in the United States wrote about 125 million opioid prescriptions in 2023. That same year, more than thirteen thousand people died from prescription opioids, and around 8.5 million people reported misusing them—meaning they took the drugs in ways not intended by their medical physician, or without a prescription at all.

Is it easily accessible?

Any medical physician can prescribe opioids, but they are controlled substances, so there are state and federal regulations that physicians must adhere to when prescribing them. In some states, opioids can also be prescribed by nurse practitioners and physician assistants.

Other considerations:

- Addressing chronic opioid use disorder or addiction goes beyond the scope of this book. The Department of Health and Human Services provides good general information on these topics (https://www.hhs.gov/opioids/index.html). To learn more about treatment for opioid use disorder, call 1-800-662-HELP (4357) or go to https://findtreatment.gov/ for help. These sources of help are anonymous, so you do not need to provide your name when contacting them.

- Although it can be prescribed legally in the United States, the majority of fentanyl used in this country is purchased illegally "on the streets." Fentanyl is particularly dangerous because is it so potent, increasing the risk of accidental overdose and death. It is often mixed with other illegal drugs so that the person taking it does not even know what they are taking.
- Methadone is an opioid that is often used to treat opioid addiction. Because it is very long acting, this drug can help prevent withdrawal symptoms and cravings.
- Buprenorphine is an opioid with mixed promoting and blocking effects on different opioid receptors. It is a potent medication that is used to treat opioid addiction because it is very long acting, prevents withdrawal symptoms, and is less likely to cause overdose than other opioids. For these same reasons, buprenorphine is sometimes used to help people taper off opioids prescribed for pain.
- The risk of opioid dependence, addiction, and death is real. If you are taking opioids, it is critically important to check in with your medical physician regularly to talk about potential harms and discuss if using fewer opioids or discontinuing their use altogether is appropriate.

Now that you have been introduced to the pain medications most often used in treating low back pain, I want to turn to Dr. Erin Krebs, whom you met in chapter 11, and Dr. Kevin Shah. Dr. Shah is the chief medical officer for Duke Primary Care. Both medical physicians have found that less is more when it comes to using prescription medications to treat low back pain. Prescription medications work only for a minority of people, and even when medication helps, the benefits are modest at best. Thus, deciding to prescribe medication for low back pain becomes a balancing act between a small potential benefit and the risk of serious side effects.

Here are some of the other lessons they have learned from conducting research and from many years of using pain medications to treat patients with low back pain.

> ***Dr. Krebs explains:***
> *When it comes to low back pain, predicting who will benefit from a particular drug before they start taking it is not possible. The severity of the pain does little to help a physician determine which medicines are most likely to be effective. People with severe pain can get significant relief from acetaminophen or capsaicin and no relief from opioids. Patients and prescribers often believe that if the drug isn't working, the answer is to prescribe more of that drug. That's one of the big problems with opioids. If prescription opioids don't work in the beginning, they're not ever going to work. If they work at first and then quit, it's time to stop them and find another treatment.*
>
> ***Dr. Shah explains:***
> *What patients want or expect can influence how a prescriber approaches prescribing pain medication. Patients often request a specific drug because they have seen an advertisement or talked to someone they know. That does not mean it will work for your specific situation. Medications are not always the right approach and sometimes can carry more risk than benefit. Watchful waiting with conservative measures will often yield better outcomes. Simply "prescribing something" is not prudent. Clinicians need to assess each individual patient for both appropriateness and risk before prescribing pain medication.*

When prescribing pain medication, Dr. Krebs always starts by asking people what they've already tried and what has worked or hasn't. If the patient hasn't tried anything yet, she begins by recommending over-the-counter topical products—patches, creams, and gels—discussed in chapter 11. These treatment approaches work for some people, she says, and have minimal downsides. For medications with a higher risk of harm, she tells patients that nothing is going to remove the pain entirely. Prescription medication is just part of the picture. The goal is to take the edge off the pain so they can focus on other things that might better address any underlying issues, such as physical activity and mindfulness. Helping patients avoid unrealistic expectations is crucial. Otherwise, they may find themselves down the path of taking more and more hazardous medications with no additional benefit.

Key Takeaways

- Prescription medications do not address the underlying causes of pain.
- Prescription medications for low back pain work only for a minority of people, and even so, the benefit is often small.
- You and your medical physician, nurse practitioner, or physician assistant must consider a balancing act between the potential benefit of a prescription medication and the risk of serious side effects.
- Because all medications carry risks, guidelines generally recommend the use of nondrug treatments for low back pain first. The WHO goes a step further and explicitly recommends against the use of most medications.
- Trial and error, along with careful monitoring of the benefits and side effects, is the best approach when trying to figure out if a specific prescription medication is right for you.

chapter 16

Interventional Procedures

This chapter focuses on commonly used interventional procedures for low back pain. They include corticosteroid injections, radiofrequency ablation, spinal cord stimulators, prolotherapy, platelet-rich plasma injections, and stem cell therapy. I will turn to specifics regarding individual interventional procedures, but several principles apply to all of them, as follows:

- Although interventional procedures are not considered surgery, they all involve either needles or small incisions to the skin and underlying tissues.
- The goal of the most commonly used interventional procedures is pain management. They do not address the underlying causes of low back pain or any Back Factors.
- Risks involved with interventional procedures vary, but the most common risks are categorized as low to moderate.
- Many guidelines do not recommend interventional procedures because they offer uncertain benefits and have known risks of harm.
- Medical physicians with specialized training perform interventional procedures. Most often these are physiatrists, physical medicine and rehabilitation specialists, neurosurgeons, interventional radiologists, and anesthesiologists.
- One quick note: Before you begin reading about interventional procedures, it might be helpful to take another look at the information included in chapter 3 about the anatomy of the spine.

Corticosteroid Injections

Corticosteroid injections, also sometimes called epidural steroid injections, are administered by a medical physician. A large needle is used to

deliver steroid medications near the spinal cord or the nerve roots coming off the spinal cord. Interlaminar corticosteroid injections are injected into the space between the vertebrae and the spinal cord. Transforaminal corticosteroid injections are injected into the area surrounding the nerve roots that exit the spinal cord. Corticosteroid injections are commonly used to treat low back pain, especially in patients experiencing pain down the back of one or both legs that is attributed to herniated discs or spinal stenosis. A 2022 study found that 14 percent of patients with chronic low back pain who saw a physician within the prior year received a corticosteroid injection. This number is far greater than the number of patients who are likely to benefit.

How does it work?

Steroid medications injected into the spine may temporarily decrease the inflammatory processes associated with a herniated disc or spinal stenosis. They may also help break apart scar tissue and temporarily increase blood flow to the area.

Is it effective?

Corticosteroid injections may decrease low back pain and physical disability for short periods. However, they do not address the underlying cause of low back pain, and there is some risk of harm. As a result, most guidelines evaluating their use recommend against them because the benefits are not worth the risks.

Is it safe?

Temporary side effects include pain, numbness, bruising, or bleeding at the injection site. Potential risks of corticosteroid injections include infection, elevated blood sugar, increased blood pressure, and, in rare cases, nerve damage.

Healthcare professionals:

Corticosteroid injections should be provided only by medical physicians who specialize in these procedures. This list includes surgeons, anesthesiologists, physiatrists (rehabilitation specialists), and physicians specializing in pain medicine. You will learn more about these medical specialists in chapter 19.

Other considerations:

- While corticosteroid injections will sometimes offer temporary pain relief to some people, they are not an effective long-term solution. As a result, they are best utilized as a short-term tool to decrease your pain enough to allow you to implement the things that can help you manage your low back pain, such as exercise and a Whole Health lifestyle.
- It would be unusual for a physician to recommend that a patient recieve more than three or four injections within a year.
- Patients whose blood sugar is regularly over 200 mg/dL or who have an A1c level greater than 8 have a higher risk of infection following corticosteroid injections.
- The cost of corticosteroid injections varies widely, ranging from $100 to $1,000.
- Most insurance plans cover all or part of the cost, but prior authorization is often required.

Radiofrequency Ablation

Radiofrequency ablation uses radiofrequency waves that generate high heat to destroy specific nerves traveling from the spine to the brain.

How does it work?

The nerves destroyed by radiofrequency ablation are no longer able to carry pain signals from the low back to the brain.

Is it effective?

Radiofrequency ablation may lead to small decreases in pain for one to three months. However, patient response is highly individualized. Although there is some disagreement among low back pain experts, most low back pain guidelines that address the use of radiofrequency ablation recommend against it because, overall, the benefits do not outweigh the potential for harm.

Is it safe?

Temporary side effects include redness or mild skin burns and changes in blood pressure. Other risks include infection, nerve damage, and potentially serious temporary increases in blood pressure. Rarely, damage to organs or tissues near the ablation site can occur.

Healthcare professionals:

Radiofrequency ablation is generally provided by medical physicians who specialize in pain management.

Other considerations:

- Like corticosteroid injections, radiofrequency ablation should only be used as a short-term tool to decrease your pain enough to allow you to implement the things that can help you manage your low back pain, such as exercise and a Whole Health lifestyle.

- The cost of radiofrequency ablation varies widely across the country, ranging from hundreds to thousands of dollars.
- Many insurance plans cover all or part of the cost, but prior authorization is almost always required.

Spinal Cord Stimulators

A spinal cord stimulator is a small device implanted under the skin near the low back. It is connected to electrodes that are inserted into the space between the vertebrae and the spinal cord. The device sends electrical impulses to the spinal cord via implanted electrodes. Spinal cord stimulators are typically used for individuals with moderate to severe chronic low back pain, especially pain associated with nerve damage, that hasn't responded well to guideline-recommended treatments.

How does it work?

Electrical impulses generated by the device stop pain signals from traveling from the spinal cord to the brain.

Is it effective?

A few studies have found that spinal cord stimulators may help some patients take fewer opioids in the short run. However, authors from a 2023 review of this literature concluded that the benefits are unlikely to outweigh the costs or the risks and recommend against their use for low back pain.

Is it safe?

Risks include infection and bleeding at the incision sites. The electrodes can move around and become misplaced, requiring additional surgery. A further risk is that the tissue forming a protective covering around the spinal cord may be cut during surgery. If this happens, it may allow the fluids in your spinal cord to leak out, causing headaches that can be severe. Rare risks include nerve damage and spinal cord injury.

Healthcare professionals:

While other physicians may implant spinal cord stimulators, the device is most likely to be implanted by an interventional pain management provider (e.g., an anesthesiologist or physical medicine and rehabilitation specialist) or a neurosurgeon.

Other considerations:

- As is true with all interventional procedures, some people benefit from this procedure while others do not. As a result, most physicians will recommend a trial run before permanently implanting the device beneath the skin. With a trial run, temporary electrodes are inserted near the spinal cord and connected to a spinal cord stimulator device that you wear under your clothing. The device is held in place by a belt placed around your waist.
- People with anxiety and depression are unlikely to be helped by spinal cord stimulators.
- The cost of spinal cord stimulators varies widely, ranging from $7,000 to $50,000.
- Most insurance plans cover all or part of the cost, but prior authorization is usually required.

Prolotherapy

Unlike the interventional procedures discussed so far, which all target nerves, prolotherapy is intended to reduce pain caused by lax or damaged ligaments and tendons. A combination of sugar, water, and a local anesthetic (e.g., lidocaine) is injected into the tissues surrounding the spine. Often, multiple injections are administered at once, with additional sessions occurring over weeks or months.

How does it work?

The primary ingredient in prolotherapy is a sugar solution. The goal of injecting this solution is to irritate damaged cells. This irritation is thought to stimulate the healing process by promoting the production of new, healthy cells.

Is it effective?

The few studies available on prolotherapy are mostly of poor quality and show conflicting results. Guidelines do not recommend prolotherapy. While some argue that multiple prolotherapy injections may have some clinical benefit, there is general agreement that a single injection is ineffective.

Is it safe?

Risks include temporary pain, numbness, bruising, or bleeding at the injection site. Infections can also occur. Rare side effects include nerve damage and spinal cord injury.

Healthcare professionals:

Prolotherapy is usually provided by healthcare professionals who specialize in pain management and are licensed to give injections.

Prolotherapy was initially classified as a complementary and integrative health treatment because the procedure was developed outside mainstream medicine. Prolotherapy is not as widely available as many other interventional procedures, but its use appears to be increasing.

Other considerations:

The cost of prolotherapy injections varies widely, ranging from $250 to $600 per session. Most insurance plans do not cover this cost as prolotherapy is considered experimental due to a lack of research on safety and effectiveness.

Platelet-Rich Plasma Injections

Platelet-rich plasma injections involve the injection of plasma and a concentrated level of platelets (up to ten times more than is found in normal blood) into damaged tendons, ligaments, and intervertebral discs. Plasma is the liquid part of your blood, made up mostly of water. Platelets are cells that help your blood clot to slow or stop bleeding. The plasma and platelets come from your own blood, so two steps are involved in preparing the injection material. The first step is to draw a small amount of blood from your arm, similar to when you have blood tests done at your medical physician's office. In the second step, a machine called a centrifuge spins the blood at a high speed to separate the plasma and platelets from the other components in your blood.

How does it work?

Platelets contain a substance called growth factor. The role of growth factor is to repair damaged cells by promoting cell growth and production. It is thought that surrounding damaged cells with higher levels of growth factor will stimulate their healing, leading to decreases in inflammation and pain sensitivity.

Is it effective?

More research is needed to evaluate the effects of platelet-rich plasma injections. I am aware of only one randomized clinical trial, which injected platelet-rich plasma into the intervertebral discs. No effect was found at one month. However, decreases in pain were observed at two months, and mild-to-moderate decreases in pain and improvements in physical function were observed at six months. Platelet-rich plasma injections are not currently recommended by low back pain guidelines, given the low number of studies available.

Is it safe?

Risks include temporary pain, numbness, bruising, or bleeding at the injection site. Infections can also occur. Rare side effects include nerve damage and spinal cord injury.

Healthcare professionals:

Platelet-rich plasma injections are generally provided by healthcare professionals who specialize in pain management and are licensed to give injections.

Other considerations:

The cost of platelet-rich plasma injections varies widely, ranging from $500 to $2,500 per session. Most insurance plans do not cover this cost, as platelet-rich plasma injections are considered experimental due to a lack of research on their safety and effectiveness. This may change as more research becomes available.

Stem Cell Treatments

Stem cells are found in many areas throughout the body. These "super-cells" can reproduce themselves and transform into entirely different cell types. The primary role of stem cells is to repair damaged cells and replenish your body with new cells as the old ones wear out. Stem cell treatments involve removing stem cells from a specific area of your body, often the hip, and then injecting them into a damaged intervertebral disc or other affected spine tissue.

How does it work?

Because stem cells can differentiate into many different cell types, they could potentially generate new intervertebral discs or other tissues of the spine. Stem cell treatments may also decrease inflammation.

Is it effective?

Stem cell treatments fall under a relatively new field called regenerative medicine. More research is needed to fully evaluate their effects. However, stem cell treatments appear to result in mild-to-moderate decreases in pain and improvements in physical function. Stem cell treatments are not currently recommended by low back pain guidelines, given the lack of evidence available.

Is it safe?

Risks include temporary pain, numbness, bruising, or bleeding at the injection site. Infections can also occur. Rare side effects include nerve damage and spinal cord injury. There is also a concern that, due to their regenerative powers, stem cells could develop into tumors or other cell abnormalities in the area where they are injected.

Healthcare professionals:

Stem cell injections are generally provided by healthcare professionals who specialize in pain management and are licensed to give injections.

Other considerations:

The cost of stem cell treatments varies widely, ranging from $5,000 to $50,000 per session. Most insurance plans do not cover this cost, as stem cell treatment for low back pain is considered to be experimental due to the lack of research on safety and effectiveness. This may change as more research becomes available.

Conversations with Clinicians and Scientists

The decision of whether or not to consider interventional procedures is a complicated one that needs to be made between you and your physician after you are fully informed of the potential for benefit versus the risk of harm. To provide more insight into the interventional procedures commonly used, I consulted three clinicians/scientists. Dr. James Eubanks is a physiatrist at the Medical University of South Carolina, and Dr. Zachary Carter is a physiatrist at Duke University School of Medicine. Dr. Jason Busse is a professor in anesthesia, faculty of health sciences at McMaster University in Hamilton, Ontario, Canada. Here are a few things they all agree on:

- Interventional procedures are not the best option for most people with low back pain.
- Nondrug treatment approaches recommended by low back pain guidelines should be tried for at least three to six months before an interventional procedure is considered.

- Interventional procedures almost always work for only a short period of time if they work at all. Patients are best served by using this short period of time while they are in less pain to engage in longer-lasting solutions, such as physical activity and other Whole Health lifestyle approaches.

Dr. Eubanks has found that patients with low back pain fall into three treatment categories. The first and largest group includes people who are best served by engaging in self-care, with added physical therapy or chiropractic care when necessary. The second group is a tiny number of patients with red flags who need surgery right away to prevent serious disease or neurological problems from getting worse. The third group is patients with chronic, complex low-back pain, undiagnosed conditions, or other illnesses that can lessen the effectiveness of self-care or self-care combined with guideline-recommended nondrug treatments. Patients in this third group are the ones Dr. Eubanks sees most often. He begins with diagnostic testing, including imaging and lab work, to rule out red flags. His next step is to discuss self-care with the patient, including bone density, weight management, and sleep optimization. He may also consider corticosteroid injections at this point, but first, he carefully considers the issues outlined above, such as the location and nature of the pain. Based on his clinical experience, he has found that the patients most likely to respond positively to interventional procedures for at least a short time are those with (1) severe pain going down one or both legs and MRI findings of a herniated disc or (2) severe pain, numbness, or tingling in the legs while walking or standing, combined with MRI confirmation of stenosis. He has also found that interventional procedures are far less helpful in patients whose pain is primarily located in the low back area, regardless of MRI findings.

Dr. Carter agrees that interventional procedures are not cures for back pain, so considering other guideline-recommended options first is critical. This reconsideration includes revisiting noninvasive treatment options even if they've failed before. He has found that even if you have tried physical therapy once and it hasn't been helpful, it is worth trying again. "Maybe it wasn't the right physical therapist," he says. "Or maybe it wasn't the right time for you." He also believes that progress in back pain management is rarely linear. "Success may also depend on taking a multimodal approach, combining different treatments, such as manual therapies and mindfulness or cognitive behavioral therapy."

Dr. Busse was the first author of a 2025 guideline on interventional procedures for chronic low back pain published in the prestigious *British Medical Journal*. He discussed the process of developing this guideline with me, explaining that nearly two dozen experts collaborated, including several individuals with primary expertise in lived experience with low back pain. Their review of the best currently available evidence led these experts to issue strong recommendations against standard interventional procedures for local or radiating chronic spine pain, including joint radiofrequency ablation, epidural injection oflocal anaesthetic, steroids, or their combination, joint-targeted injection of local anaesthetic, steroids, or their combination, intramuscular injection of local anaesthetic with or without steroids, and dorsal root ganglion radiofrequency. They found no evidence of benefit across any subgroup of patients and concluded that interventional procedures should be administered only in clinical trials until evidence supports their use in practice.

Key Takeaways

- Interventional procedures for low back pain vary widely in their potential risks, benefits, and costs.
- Interventional procedures do not address the underlying causes of low back pain
- Relief from interventional procedures is usually temporary at best.
- Everyone has a different perspective on what potential benefits are worth the risk of harm. This is a choice you will have to make for yourself, in consultation with your physician, after becoming fully aware of the potential risks involved for you as an individual.
- Finding a physician who will talk to you about the risks and benefits of interventional procedures is essential. These discussions should also include information on the full range of other treatments available, including nondrug approaches.

chapter 17

Surgery for Low Back Pain

If you are considering surgery to address your low back pain, read this chapter carefully and discuss any concerns with your surgeon before you make a final decision. Sometimes surgery for low back pain is absolutely the right choice. Most often, it is not. With other treatments for low back pain, there is room to evaluate the benefits and side effects of different options. If one thing doesn't work, you can always add another therapy or switch to something else. Surgery is different. It is associated with a significantly higher risk of complications or poor outcomes than most other treatments. You may feel stiff and sore after spinal manipulation or an exercise session, but with surgery, you are making permanent changes to the spine and its surrounding tissues. Surgery comes with high physical and emotional costs—recovery from the procedure itself can take several months and often longer. Finally, surgery is highly personalized. This means that research focused on whether treatments are safe and effective on average is less helpful in guiding individual people in the right direction. In other words, what works for your neighbor down the street may not work for you.

I'll start by explaining what is known about spine surgery for low back pain in general and walk you through the basics of several standard surgical procedures. Next, I will share insights gained from conversations with three exceptional spine surgeons who have performed thousands of surgeries on patients with low back pain throughout their careers.

Surgery 101

Surgeries for low back pain fall into two basic categories: (1) treatments for an acute medical emergency, and (2) everything else. An acute surgical emergency is a condition in which a delay in treatment could result in significant harm to the patient. Examples include some of the red flag conditions that we discussed in chapter 3: progressive weakness in the legs, cancer, infection, and loss of bowel or bladder control. While rare, these causes of low back pain need to be addressed immediately if they are present. The overwhelming majority of surgeries for low back pain fall into the "everything else" category. While these "everything else" surgeries are sometimes called elective, that term is misleading. Elective does not mean the surgery is frivolous or unneeded. It simply refers to any surgery that is not a medical emergency.

Risks Versus Benefits of Spine Surgery

Risks

The list of potential risks associated with spine surgery is long. These risks include ending up worse after the surgery than you were before, increased odds of needing future surgeries, and the real possibility of opioid use disorder or addiction. Spine surgery is also a costly, major life event. It requires significant preparation and recovery time with no guarantee that you will be able to return to pre–low back pain work or home life.

Many people considering surgery for low back pain struggle to put these abstract risks into perspective. Let me give you a few numbers to help you get there.

- Catastrophic nerve injuries are rare following spine surgery for low back pain, but they do occur. Examples include permanent leg weakness, numbness, bowel or bladder issues, and even paralysis. The estimated risk of one of these events is between .13 percent and .25 percent for a discectomy, .5 percent for a spinal fusion, and 2 percent for an open laminectomy.
- About 15 percent of people who get surgery for chronic low back pain have another surgery within five years. That

number is higher for revision discectomy (18 percent) than lumbar fusion (6 percent).

- Up to 40 percent of people who have spine surgery for low back pain have persistent pain afterward.

- More than 60 percent of people on workers' compensation who get spinal surgery for chronic primary low back pain are not working two years later.

- As many as 15 percent of surgical patients end up with persistent spinal pain, meaning their pain and disability are significantly worse following the surgery.

- A few years ago, it was difficult to pick up a newspaper without reading something about the opioid crisis—and justifiably so. You learned about opioids in chapter 15. Relevant to this discussion, a 2020 study found that 63 percent of people undergoing lumbar spine surgery were still taking opioids more than ninety days later.

- Even if your spine surgery goes perfectly, it is still a significant life event that requires considerable planning. Making sure you are as healthy as possible before surgery will lower the risk of complications. You will have a period when you need people to care for you, rather than the other way around. For some, this means planning for temporary help and ensuring that the people in your life who depend on you for care (e.g., children or parents) are covered. You will need to take time off work if you are employed.

- Lastly, spine surgery can cost $100,000 or more, so it's also important to discuss the financial implications with your health insurance plan and ensure you understand the costs.

Benefits

I mentioned earlier that evaluating surgical procedures from a research perspective, including spine surgery, is challenging. The best way to collect evidence on the safety and effectiveness of surgery for low back pain would be to conduct a sham-controlled study where researchers compare real surgery to a sham, that is, pretend, surgery. Due to the potential risk to those who would receive no benefit, this rarely occurs. Instead, researchers tend to compare two different surgical procedures or to compare surgery with a nonsurgical treatment, such as rehabilitation or other nonsurgical approaches.

The results of these studies show that the long-term benefits of surgery for most people are relatively small compared to nonsurgical options. Some studies have found no benefit. The people most likely to experience improvements in pain and disability after surgery are those who have (1) chronic, moderate to severe radiculopathy related to a herniated disc or other specific finding in the spine, and (2) have not responded well to other guideline-recommended, nonsurgical treatments. However, even in these cases, patient outcomes are often no better in the long run. It is essential to weigh the potential short- and long-term benefits of surgery against the risk of harm. Having the right information to help you make that decision is critical. Here are a few important details about the surgeries most commonly used for low back pain.

Surgical Procedures Used in Treating Low Back Pain

The most common surgical procedures used to treat low back pain are laminectomy, discectomy, and spinal fusion. It may be helpful to review chapter 3 on spinal anatomy before reading further.

Laminectomy and Decompression

Remember the odd-shaped bones in your spine, called vertebrae, discussed in chapter 3? They protect your spinal cord and the nerves attached to the spinal cord. The spinous processes are the bony bumps you feel as you run your hand down the middle of your back. The lamina connect the spinous processes to the rest of the vertebra and protect the spinal cord and nerves coming off the spinal cord. Injury or degeneration here can cause compression of the nerves in the spine. When this happens, the spinal nerves are less able to supply the muscles of the low back with the necessary amount of oxygen and nutrients needed for normal movement. This can result in leg pain, weakness, or numbness. With a laminectomy, the surgeon removes the lamina to leave more room for your spinal cord and/or spinal nerves. This process is called decompression.

With an open laminectomy, in addition to removing the lamina, the surgeon removes the spinous process, the ligaments attaching the spinous processes, and the muscles attached to the back of the vertebra. For a minimally invasive laminectomy, the surgeon removes only the lamina, cutting through fewer muscles in the process. A laminectomy is called a laminotomy when only part of the lamina is removed.

Discectomy and Decompression

Discectomy is another decompression method, used primarily to address intervertebral disc herniations. With a standard discectomy, the surgeon first performs a laminectomy to access the intervertebral disc in question. They then remove the part of the disc that is putting pressure on the spinal cord or spinal nerves. With a microdiscectomy, the surgeon uses a microscope to make smaller incisions. This procedure is considered less invasive because it affects fewer muscles and other back tissues. An endoscopic discectomy uses a tiny camera and small surgical instruments, resulting in a smaller incision and less disruption to the tissues surrounding the spine.

Spinal Fusion

As its name suggests, spinal fusion involves fusing two or more vertebrae into one unit. The vertebrae are permanently held together using either real bone (grafts) or an artificial bone-like material. The newly conjoined vertebrae are screwed in place so that they stay together while the bone graft or artificial bone hardens. Spinal fusions are most commonly used when the intervertebral disc becomes thin due to arthritis or other causes and is no longer able to provide adequate cushioning between two vertebrae. This surgery is also used to treat scoliosis and spine fractures.

Spinal fusion can lead to a condition known as adjacent segment disease. Fusing two or more vertebrae stops normal spine movement in the area where the surgery occurs. While that might correct a problem at that particular segment, it also puts a lot of additional pressure on the spine above and below the fused area. That pressure can cause arthritis or degeneration of the bones and soft tissues, leading to increased pain and disability in the long run. The result is sometimes more surgery. Among surgeons, there's a growing awareness that spinal fusion leads to adjacent segment disease too often. However, newer surgical techniques referred to as "motion sparing" may help prevent these situations. Fusion surgery is evolving at such a rapid rate that it is smart to seek more than one opinion about the best option for you before going down this route.

In summary, multiple surgical options are used to address low back pain. The goal of each is to relieve nerve pressure or stabilize the spine. While spine surgery can sometimes provide short-term relief—particularly for nerve-related pain—for many people, the long-term benefits are modest at best. These benefits must be weighed against the sometimes substantial risks involved, including the possibility of additional surgeries down the line. Also, the field of spinal surgery is constantly changing. New, less invasive techniques offer hope of better outcomes with less risk involved. You may want to talk with more than one surgeon to get multiple opinions on your options. Ultimately, the decision on whether or not to have surgery rests on your shoulders. You want to be as informed as possible when making that decision.

Actions You Can Take to Optimize Your Surgery Outcomes

If you do decide to have surgery, it's helpful to know what actions you can take to make a good result more likely. Getting ready for surgery is similar to preparing to run a marathon. Your success depends on the actions you take to prepare yourself in advance—physically, emotionally, and socially. Many of the actions required are consistent with taking the Whole Health approach discussed in chapters 5 and 6. Such preparation requires self-empowerment, motivation, and resilience, but it is well worth the effort. You will be more prepared for surgery, leading to fewer complications before and after surgery and a better chance of achieving your surgical goals of less pain and improved functioning afterward. You might even find that you no longer feel that you need surgery as a result of this preparation.

- Be mindful of your body mass index. Patients with a body mass index above 35 have a higher risk of surgical complications and poorer surgical outcomes.
- If you have high blood pressure, do everything possible to lower it. Hypertension is associated with worse surgical outcomes overall.
- Do everything possible to get your diabetes under control. Surgical wounds take longer to heal when blood sugar levels are too high.
- Stop smoking at least six weeks before surgery. Smoking increases infection rates and decreases the likelihood of a successful fusion.
- Consider mindfulness and cognitive behavioral therapy to address mental health issues. People experiencing anxiety, depression, fear avoidance, and ONTs are more likely to have poor surgical outcomes.
- Work on your cardiac health. People with heart problems are more likely to experience complications following surgery.

- Talk with your physician about the need to change your use of prescription and nonprescription medications, as well as any nutritional supplements you are taking. Blood thinners can lead to increased bleeding during and after surgery, while high levels of narcotic medication usage before surgery can make it harder to control postoperative pain.
- Develop or activate a strong social support system and have a solid plan in place to get the help you need during the postoperative recovery period. This will lead to a shorter recovery period.
- Be as physically active as possible before surgery. One of the most important factors to consider when recovering from back surgery is maintaining mobility. If you're not mobile to start with, then recovery becomes much more difficult, even when the surgery is done perfectly.
- Eat healthy. Even if your body mass index is below 35, poor nutrition from eating foods that are high in sugar and other empty calories can make surgical outcomes worse. Abnormal albumin and pure prealbumin levels can affect wound healing and overall response to surgery.
- Do whatever you can to increase your bone density if it is lower than normal, especially if you are a postmenopausal woman. Poor bone density is associated with worse surgical outcomes.

Three Spine Surgeons' Takes on Surgery for Low Back Pain

To provide you with the best available information on spine surgery, I turned to three of the best spine surgeons I know. Dr. Oren Gottfried is a professor of neurosurgery, a professor in the Department of Orthopaedic Surgery, and vice chair for clinical and quality outcomes at Duke University School of Medicine. Dr. Gottfried specializes in the surgical management of complex lumbar and sacral spinal disorders related to arthritis or degenerative disease, deformity, tumors, and trauma. Dr. Muhammad Abd-El-Barr is a professor of neurosurgery, associate professor in the Department of Orthopaedics, and chief of endoscopic spine surgery at Duke University School of Medicine. Dr. Abd-El-Barr treats patients with spinal stenosis, spondylolisthesis, scoliosis, herniated discs, and spine tumors, often using the minimally invasive techniques I touched on earlier. Dr. Joe Minchew is an associate professor in the Department of Orthopaedic Surgery and an associate professor in neurosurgery at Duke University School of Medicine. Dr. Minchew specializes in lumbar disc herniations, spinal stenosis, vertebral compression fractures, spondylolisthesis, and spine injections.

These physicians have spent a lot of time in the operating room. They have also encouraged many patients not to have surgery. Here are a few things they wish more people knew about spine surgery for low back pain.

1. Surgery is not appropriate for most people with low back pain.

Examples of when surgery is appropriate include severe spinal stenosis, spinal instability, deformity, and the red flag symptoms already discussed. Another is radiculopathy in one or both legs that does not respond to three to six months of nonoperative treatments. According to Dr. Gottfried, "Some people believe surgery is the default when nothing else has worked. This is not true. Surgery should only be considered if the person is experiencing a high level of pain and disability that significantly impacts their lives, and every single possible nonoperative conservative treatment has been tried. Their symptoms and imaging must also match a problem that is treatable with surgery."

Dr. Minchew agrees. "Unless you have a structurally correctable problem, such as a spondylolisthesis or a progressive scoliotic deformity," he says, "I don't think there's ever a great indication for low back pain surgery. The results are variable at best."

Patients with multilevel age-related disc degeneration or arthritis will probably not get the response to surgery that they are hoping for. The same is true for people facing unaddressed mental health issues, people with high levels of life stress, chronic narcotics users, or people who are unable to work. People with chronic diffuse pain syndromes like fibromyalgia and complex regional pain syndromes in addition to low back pain are also more likely to have poor surgical outcomes.

2. What to consider when you are offered the "latest and greatest" spine surgery techniques.

New surgical techniques are constantly being developed. How do you know how far to go down the path of the latest and greatest? Dr. Abd-El-Barr says this question is tricky. On the one hand, new surgical techniques might lead to better outcomes and shorter recovery periods. On the other hand, there are examples of "fad" surgeries ultimately abandoned because they were not effective or were associated with too many complications. If your surgeon suggests a new surgical technique, Dr. Abd-El-Barr recommends you ask a lot of questions. Here are some suggestions. "Have there been any published studies on the outcomes versus risks following this surgery?" "What are the benefits at six months, one year, two years, and ten years?" You will also want to consider the surgeon's experience and expertise with any new approach. "Ask how many of these procedures the surgeon has done," advises Dr. Abd-El-Barr. "If the surgeon appears uncomfortable answering all your questions, that's a red flag." Ask for a referral to someone else or seek a second opinion from a different surgeon.

3. Your surgeon might recommend against surgery. Pay attention to that advice.

Surgeons have hard conversations with patients all the time. However, it might surprise you to learn that their most difficult conversations are not when they have to break the news that a complex surgery is needed immediately. The hard conversations are with people in a lot of pain who are not the right candidates for surgery. People who are desperate to find a way out of their low back pain. They come to the surgeon's office because someone—often another healthcare professional—told them surgery was the answer. Dr. Abd-El-Barr recommends several key points to keep in mind if this happens to you. "For the most part, surgeons love to operate. If a surgeon is hesitant, it should make you think twice. Ask yourself, 'Why is this person who loves to do surgery telling me I'm not a good candidate?' Keep in mind that the surgeon has your best interests in mind and has a limited set of tools. There are only certain things that we can do, and if we don't feel that what's in our toolbox will help you, please take that to heart."

Dr. Gottfried notes that you may have conditions other than your low back pain that make surgery more dangerous or less likely to succeed in your case. If so, ask your surgeon whether there are any steps you can take to make surgery a better option in the future. "If I were picking a surgeon," he says, "it would be someone willing to take on the long-term commitment of working with me to decrease my low back pain and disability, even if surgery never happens."

Dr. Minchew says that when a surgeon recommends against surgery, it is essential to pay attention to two things: what the surgeon is saying and what the surgeon is not saying.

Dr. Minchew explains:

The surgeon is telling you that they don't think that you'll benefit from surgery. They have discussed your symptoms with you, reviewed your imaging studies, and don't see a problem that can reliably be addressed by surgery, given the, albeit low, risks. They are saying they don't want to do anything that could make you worse. The surgeon is NOT saying that they don't believe that you have pain or serious difficulties. The surgeon is NOT saying that you're destined to live with your low back the way it is now or that your pain and disability will get worse. The surgeon is NOT saying that there are no effective treatments available.

4. Successful recovery from spine surgery requires planning.

Dr. Minchew emphasizes the need for a concrete plan to ensure you have the necessary support after surgery. If you plan to go home right after surgery, arranging for help with the basic activities of daily living is essential. Tasks such as meal preparation, toileting, and transportation to and from postoperative medical physician's visits can be challenging without support. If the surgeon thinks there is even a possibility that you will need to spend time in a rehabilitation center or a nursing home afterward, ensure this is arranged in advance. Discussing all possible scenarios with your surgeon in advance is essential. You need to have realistic expectations about how you are likely to feel after the surgery and what level of assistance you may require as a result. Such decisions depend on how well your body tolerates the surgery. Also, keep in mind that after surgery, your surgeon does not decide whether you can go home or need to consider a nursing home or a rehabilitation center. The nurses, physical therapists, and case managers at the hospital will be the ones who are addressing those issues.

5. Recovering from surgery takes time and is directly related to your presurgery preparation/wellness.

As Dr. Abd-El-Barr points out, surgery is an assault on your physical being, your social being, and your psychological being. It is crucial to be prepared for that. He views surgery as taking one step backward to go two steps forward. The time it takes to recover depends on the type of surgery and your overall health before the surgery. "With some surgeries," says Dr. Abd-El-Barr, "you will feel better very quickly. With more complicated surgeries, it can take up to a year to fully recover. Addressing modifiable risk factors helps support a faster recovery, since you have a healthier body to start with. So does the use of newer, more minimally invasive techniques."

Dr. Minchew agrees that recovery time depends on the procedure. He says that with microdiscectomy and microdecompression procedures, most people can return to daily activities within two weeks. Within four to six weeks, you can resume most activities, including driving. For the best post-surgical results, avoid sports like tennis, golf, basketball, and skiing for twelve weeks. For more complex surgeries, recovery times can vary significantly: It may take four to six weeks to feel normal, three months to resume exercise and similar physical activities, and up to nine months to fully recover.

Dr. Gottfried advises listening to your surgeon regarding how long recovery will take and developing very concrete milestones or goals along the way. Then write those milestones down on a calendar. This tactic will help you stay on track and prevent discouragement along the way. He also advises against trying to do too much too fast after surgery. "Some of my patients try to do too much when they begin to feel a little bit better," he says. "This can cause postsurgical complications that could have been avoided."

6. Surgery for low back pain never comes with a pain-free guarantee.

"You are going to have pain after surgery," Dr. Minchew says. "We will do everything we can to minimize that pain, but there is no safe dose of drugs we can offer that will make it go away entirely." Even his patients who have had tremendous results will admit that they still, at times, have low back pain. A more realistic expectation is less pain and better functioning with fewer medications.

7. Not all surgeries are successful.

Dr. Abd-El-Barr recommends evaluating the success of your surgery at the six-month mark by asking yourself, "Am I better, the same, or worse than I was six months ago?" Filling out the Personal Health Inventory found in chapter 6, before surgery and then at three months, six months, and twelve months afterward, can help you answer this question. If your low back pain worsens six months to a year after surgery, Dr. Abd-El-Barr recommends discussing the potential reasons with your surgeon.

Choose Your Treatment Approaches

You have reached the end of part 2 of this book. As a result, you are familiar with the wide range of treatments most commonly used to treat low back pain. Now it is time to apply that knowledge to your specific low back pain situation. Start by reviewing the Back Factors you listed at the end of chapter 4. Then use the Find Your Treatments Diagram in figure 9 on the next page to identify which treatment approaches are the best match with those Back Factors. Save your treatment options list. It will be helpful as you develop your Take Your Back Back Action Plan in chapter 22.

List your treatment options here:

Treatment Approach #1 ______________________

Treatment Approach #2 ______________________

Treatment Approach #3 ______________________

Treatment Approach #4 ______________________

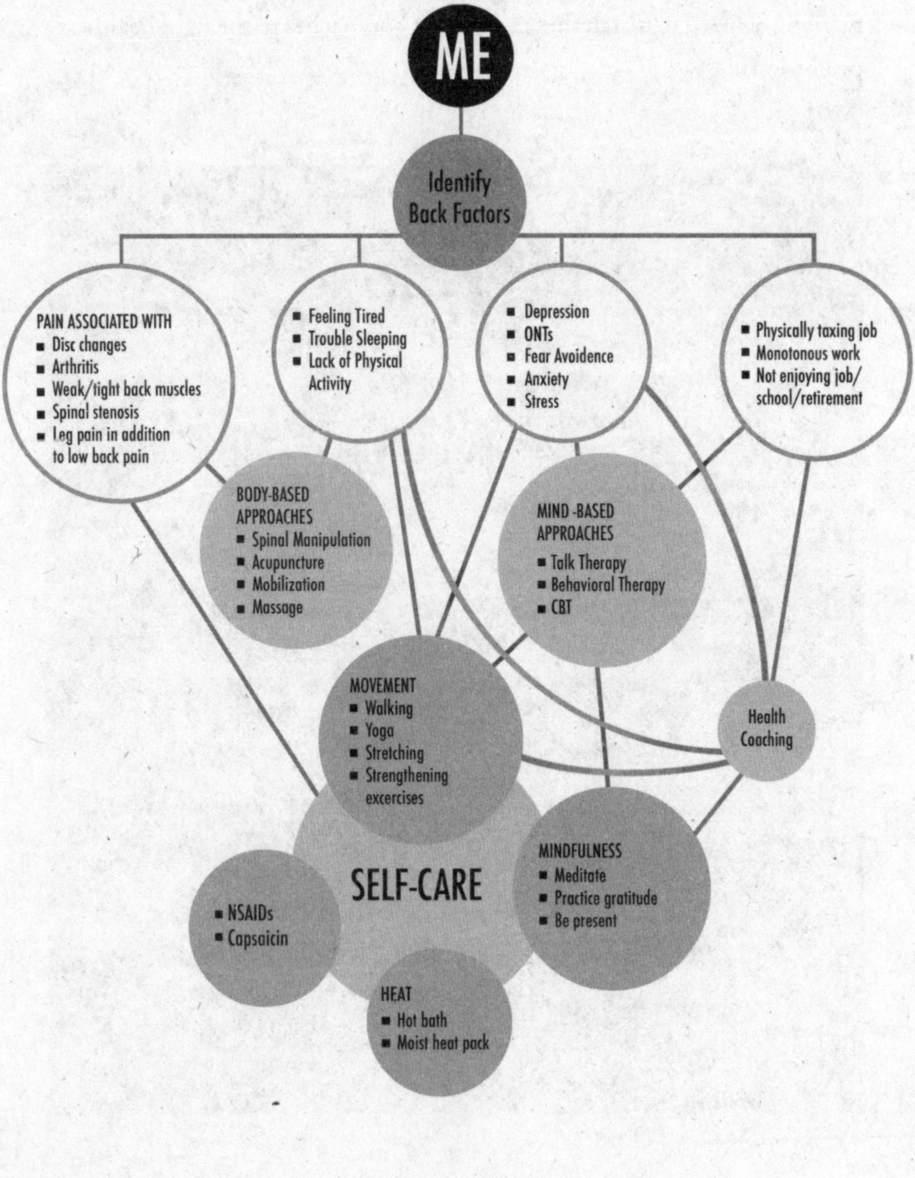
ME
Identify Back Factors
PAIN ASSOCIATED WITH
Disc changes
Arthritis
Weak/tight back muscles
Spinal stenosis
Leg pain in addition to low back pain
Feeling Tired
Trouble Sleeping
Lack of Physical Activity
Depression
ONTs
Fear Avoidence
Anxiety
Stress
Physically taxing job
Monotonous work
Not enjoying job/school/retirement
BODY-BASED APPROACHES
Spinal Manipulation
Acupuncture
Mobilization
Massage
MIND-BASED APPROACHES
Talk Therapy
Behavioral Therapy
CBT
MOVEMENT
Walking
Yoga
Stretching
Strengthening excercises
Health Coaching
SELF-CARE
NSAIDs
Capsaicin
MINDFULNESS
Meditate
Practice gratitude
Be present
HEAT
Hot bath
Moist heat pack

Figure 9

Next up in *Take Your Back Back* is part 3, where you will find the information you need to match these treatment approaches to the right healthcare professional(s).

Key Takeaways

- Elective surgery is rarely the answer to low back pain and should be considered only after guideline-recommended treatments have been tried.
- Spine surgery for low back pain may not be successful and carries significant risks, including the possibility of serious harm and long recovery times.
- Surgery is a a very individualized approach, meaning that what works for one patient may not work for another.
- The decision to have surgery is a big one. Make sure you and your family members have asked every question you can think of beforehand. If you are not satisfied with the answers you receive, consider finding another surgeon.
- If you do opt for surgery, plan for your surgery as if you were preparing for a marathon. Your success depends a great deal on the actions you take to prepare yourself in advance—physically, emotionally, and socially.

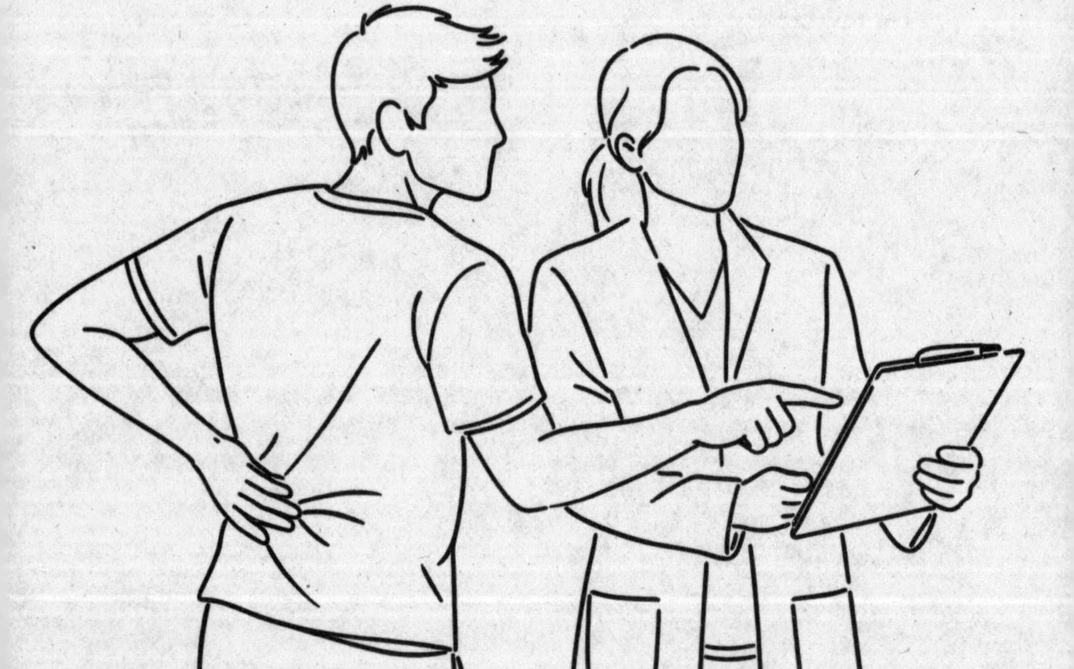

Part Three

Taking Action

chapter 18

Finding the Right Healthcare Professional

It is critically important to make the right choice when it comes to choosing the professional (or professionals) best able to help you during your low back pain journey. Given the many options, this can be a daunting task. In the next few chapters, you will find information about the required training, credentialing, treatment approaches, and other relevant details regarding a wide range of clinicians and other professionals. This chapter describes why you might want to consider either a physical therapist or a doctor of chiropractic first for most low back pain. You will also learn more about mental healthcare professionals and when they can be a crucial part of your healthcare team. Chapter 19 provides information on medical professionals and their role in caring for people with low back pain. Chapter 20 focuses on trained professionals such as health coaches who, while not low back pain experts, may be able to help you achieve your overall Whole Health goals.

One thing to keep in mind: The role of any healthcare professional is not to single-handedly "fix" your low back pain. Rather, they are there to support you in managing your low back pain and achieving your Whole Health goals.

What to Expect from Any Healthcare Professional Helping You Manage Your Low Back Pain

Before diving into any specifics, review the following few key principles that should be true for all healthcare professionals, regardless of their training and credentials.

- They work with you to identify as many Back Factors as possible, rather than focusing on a narrow medical diagnosis. Alice Kongsted, PhD, professor at the Department of Sports Science and

Clinical Biomechanics at the University of Southern Denmark, explains this well. "Be skeptical if you have chronic low back pain and your clinician gives you a simple diagnosis: a weak muscle, a muscle spasm, a misalignment of the spine, or a joint dysfunction. I understand how appealing that can be when you have been experiencing low back pain for a long time. Finally, you have found somebody who can tell you what is wrong and what one treatment will work. But most long-lasting low back pain problems are more complex than that." Be equally skeptical of someone who tells you that there is no hope, that you have to learn to live with chronic, disabling pain. As Dr. Kongsted says, "While there may not be a simple cure or one solution for your low back pain, you can learn ways to manage both the pain and your life. A skilled clinician can help you discover changes you can make that allow you to reengage in things that you value."

- You trust their advice.
- They help you identify solutions for your low back pain that fit with your experiences and needs.
- They have an excellent reputation among their patients, their staff, their community, and other healthcare professionals.
- They are patient-centered. This means treating you with respect, listening to what you have to say, and ensuring you are an essential partner in the decision-making process.
- They have the skills required to evaluate your condition and then either provide necessary treatments or refer you to a different healthcare professional who can.
- They diagnose health conditions in the context of their expertise and your overall health and wellness.

- They work with you as a partner in setting up your health goals, developing care plans based on those goals, and providing the encouragement and help you need to fully engage in self-care.
- They support your Whole Health approach. This includes discussing your lifestyle, work habits, and physical activity levels with you.
- They help you identify treatment approaches tailored to your specific needs, based on an evidence-based approach. This means they follow the latest research and guideline recommendations.
- You walk away from your first appointment with a clear understanding of the recommended course of care, the potential risks and benefits involved with any treatments, what outcomes you can expect in both the short and long term, and the costs involved.

Some of these characteristics are easy to identify up front, while others may require a visit or two to evaluate. If you feel like you are not connecting with a person or that something just isn't right, trust your gut. Consider seeing a different healthcare professional.

Doctor of Chiropractic or Physical Therapist?

Doctors of chiropractic and physical therapists who follow guideline-based best practices and focus on low back pain are among the best healthcare professionals to consider first when starting on your low back pain journey. Both professions are trained as first-contact clinicians, and studies show that the treatment approaches they deliver are effective and can result in fewer invasive procedures/surgeries, adverse drug events, and opioid prescriptions, usually at a lower cost. Here are some of the similarities and differences between these two professions.

In general, evidence-based chiropractors and physical therapists who treat patients with low back pain:

- Start a first visit with a detailed history and examination to learn your low back pain story and either diagnose your condition or help you determine what Back Factors might be contributing to your pain.
- Have experience working with low back pain patients.
- Are expert in delivering guideline-recommended treatment approaches such as exercise instruction and manual therapies.
- Provide self-care recommendations and advice.
- Can refer you to other healthcare professionals if needed. In fact, because chiropractors and physical therapists tend to see their patients several times within a short period, they are well positioned to identify patients who are not responding to their care as expected. As a result, they can make timely specialist referrals when needed.
- Can provide support during the inevitable ups and downs common with chronic pain. This support may include treatment plan changes, additional diagnostic testing, and appropriate referrals.
- Are considered first-contact healthcare professionals in all fifty states. This means that you do not need a referral to see them, and they are trained to assess and manage a large range of spine-related patient conditions.
- Are covered by most insurance plans. Remember to always contact your insurance company regarding coverage before making an appointment with any healthcare professional. More about this in chapter 21.

Although there can be many similarities in the care offered by chiropractors and physical therapists, there are a few key differences that may help you decide which is right for you:

- If spinal manipulation is one of the treatment approaches that best matches your Back Factors, consider seeing a chiropractor first. As a rule, chiropractors typically focus on spinal manipulation and other manual therapies. Not all physical therapists have extensive training in manual therapies.
- If exercise is your best Back Factor match, consider seeing a physical therapist first. Strengthening exercises are a core tool in the physical therapist's tool bag, while exercise advice is often considered a supportive approach among chiropractors.
- If you receive your healthcare coverage through Medicare or Medicaid, you may end up paying less out of your pocket with a physical therapist than a chiropractor. This is due to outdated payment policies, which you will learn more about in chapter 21.
- Chiropractors are licensed to diagnose patient conditions and can refer you directly to medical specialists or for imaging or other diagnostic testing.
- Physical therapists can identify levels of impairment and physical limitations, but diagnosing medical conditions is outside their scope of practice. In addition, they are rarely able to order diagnostic testing directly. However, they can notify your primary care physician that you may need these services.
- Although physical therapists are technically first-access clinicians in every state, many health insurance plans and health systems require a physician referral or review of the care plan by a medical physician to either begin or continue care.

- Physical therapists are most likely to be integrated into healthcare systems, and your medical physician will almost always be able to refer you to a physical therapist whom they have worked with in the past.

Doctors of Chiropractic (Chiropractor/DC)

Up to 18 percent of US adults visit a chiropractor each year, and about 50 percent see a chiropractor at some point in their lives. Most chiropractors focus on treating patients with spine-related disorders, including low back pain. As a result, they are well trained to diagnose low back pain, provide guideline-recommended treatments, and help patients to actively manage their condition. Chiropractors also commonly help patients develop personalized care plans that emphasize self-care and make referrals to medical specialists or other healthcare professionals when needed. Most insurance plans cover chiropractic care to some extent.

Treatment approaches:

Manual therapies with an emphasis on spinal manipulation, exercise advice and instruction, patient education, therapeutic ultrasound, laser treatment, electrical muscle stimulation, superficial heat, and nutritional advice. Some chiropractors are also trained in acupuncture.

Training and credentials:

To practice in the United States, chiropractors must complete four years of doctoral-level training at an educational institution accredited by the Council on Chiropractic Education, in addition to at least three years of undergraduate education, and receive their doctor of chiropractic degree. They must also pass four exams administered by the National Board of Chiropractic Examiners, as well as any other tests required by individual states, to become licensed. Annual continuing education is required.

Finding the right person:

When choosing the right chiropractor, several factors come into play. Below is some guidance on making that decision.

In 2012, the American Board of Internal Medicine spearheaded the Choosing Wisely Program. Their goal was to help decrease the use of low-value care—medical tests and procedures that don't work very well, have a significant risk of harm, and/or are expensive. In response, more than eighty healthcare societies developed profession-specific lists of five tests, treatments, and procedures that are either overused or inconsistent with research and guideline recommendations. Below is the list that the American Chiropractic Association developed for chiropractors and their patients:

- Avoid routine spinal imaging in the absence of clear clinical indicators for patients with acute low back pain of less than six weeks' duration.
- Do not perform repeat imaging to monitor patients' progress.
- Avoid protracted use of passive or palliative physical therapeutic modalities for low back pain disorders unless they support the goal(s) of an active treatment plan.
- Do not provide long-term pain management without psychosocial screening or assessment.
- Do not prescribe lumbar supports or braces for the long-term treatment or prevention of low back pain.

It should be emphasized that the tests and procedures in this list are sometimes the wise choice. However, they should not be done "routinely" on every patient. If your chiropractor recommends any items on this list, ask why and ensure the answer addresses your specific Back Factors and overall clinical circumstances.

Dr. Louis Sportelli is the current president of the National Chiropractic Mutual Insurance Company Research Foundation. I first met Dr. Sportelli while I was a chiropractic student, when I drove from Minneapolis to Chicago to hear him give a lecture on chiropractic professionalism. In addition to the characteristics described earlier that apply to all clinicians, there are several things that would cause him to proceed with caution when choosing a chiropractor:

- Seeking payment in advance for multiple future visits.
- Charging considerably more than the average rate for the services provided.
- Not clearly explaining the causes of your healthcare condition or why the recommended treatment approach should help.
- Trying to "sell" you something, be it multiple sessions of spinal manipulation, nutritional supplements, or other devices or treatments where the product or service can only be obtained from that facility.
- Giving what sounds like a well-rehearsed sales pitch rather than a personalized care plan.
- Saying things that frighten you, especially if the answer to your frightening condition is a large number of chiropractic treatments. For example, you are told that degeneration of the spine or the curves in your spine will get worse if you do not receive a large number of chiropractic visits.
- Using words or language that you don't understand. "This is not communication," says Dr. Sportelli. "This is an attempt to either impress or scare you."

Cost:

The cost of consulting a chiropractor varies depending on the services provided. A first visit may cost several hundred dollars, while follow-up visits tend to cost $40–$100. As stated earlier, most insurance plans cover chiropractic care to some extent, but large co-pays and denial of some services are common. Be sure to check with your insurance company before your first visit to avoid surprises. Usually, the chiropractic office can assist you in this process. You will find more on addressing payment challenges for guideline-recommended care for low back pain in chapter 21.

Other considerations:

The frequency of chiropractor visits varies based on your underlying condition. However, you should be able to tell within four to six visits whether chiropractic care is helping you manage your low back pain. The need for additional care should be determined on an individual basis based on your underlying condition, age, occupation, and lifestyle.

Physical Therapists (PTs/DPTs)

In the United States, approximately 50 million people see a physical therapist each year. This number increases with age—about 50 percent of US adults see a physical therapist at some point in their lives. Physical therapists are integrated into most health systems across the country, and their care is covered at least to some extent by nearly all health insurance plans.

Physical therapists treat patients with a broad range of conditions, including people recovering from stroke, heart attacks, or trauma and those with musculoskeletal disorders. Their primary focus is rehabilitation and addressing physical disability/pain. Many physical therapists specialize in a specific area, such as postsurgical rehabilitation or stroke recovery. If you choose a physical therapist as your first-contact clinician, consider someone with specific expertise in managing low back pain.

Treatment approaches:

Supervised strengthening exercise, physical activity, exercise advice/instruction, patient education, therapeutic ultrasound, electrical muscle stimulation, self-empowerment strategies, nutritional advice, and sometimes manual therapies and dry needling.

Training and credentials:

All physical therapists graduating in the United States today from an academic institution approved by the Commission on Accreditation in Physical Therapy Education (CAPTE) must have a doctor of physical therapy degree (DPT). However, physical therapists with either a bachelor's or a master's degree who graduated before this requirement was implemented may practice under the umbrella of their original credentials (PT). Physical Therapy Assistants (PTAs) frequently work closely with physical therapists in providing patient care. PTAs need to graduate from a two-year training program accredited by the CAPTE.

Finding the right person:

Trevor Lentz, PT, PhD, MPH, associate professor of orthopaedic surgery at Duke University, believes you can quickly determine whether a physical therapist is the right person for you. He advises paying attention to how you feel as you walk out of the physical therapist's office after your initial visit. "There should be a sense of optimism, a feeling that this healthcare professional understands you as a person and how low back pain is affecting your life," he says. "You should feel that you have more information about the factors contributing to your pain and have a clear sense of what needs to happen next, including what you can do on your own to address your pain." Dr. Lentz cautions that it may then take two or three visits to determine if the treatment approach recommended by the physical therapist is right for you. "Sometimes," Dr. Lentz says, "it takes a little time for the physical therapist to understand what will work best for you as an individual patient." There is some trial and error involved, especially at first.

Here are a few things that would cause Dr. Lentz to proceed with caution when seeking care from a physical therapist:

- Multiple visits in a row where you receive only electrical muscle stimulation, therapeutic ultrasound, and hot or cold packs. Treatment should focus primarily on exercise, Whole Health or self-management strategies, and manual therapies.
- Feeling bounced around among various physical therapy providers (PTs, PTAs, aides, etc.) without regular check-ins with your primary physical therapist. This pattern can make it challenging to build the kind of relationships that help facilitate positive outcomes for low back pain.
- A physical therapist who does more talking at you than listening to what you have to say, or who doesn't give you plenty of time to make sure that all of your questions are answered to your satisfaction.
- Failing to provide clear instructions on recommended self-care.

Costs:

The cost of consulting a physical therapist varies depending on the services provided. A first visit may cost several hundred dollars, while follow-up visits tend to cost considerably less. Physical therapy is likely to be covered by health insurance to some extent, but often, large co-payments are required. Some health systems and insurance plans require a referral from a medical physician to see a physical therapist, typically after a specified number of days or visits have been completed.

Other considerations:

According to Dr. Cook, whom you met in chapter 11, affiliation with an academic institution or holding a doctoral-level degree doesn't necessarily predict whether a physical therapist is right for you. What he believes matters most is the physical therapists' experience and abilities in treating low back pain, as well as their relationships with other healthcare professionals, including physiatrists, primary care physicians, and surgeons. He recommends the American Academy of Orthopaedic Manual Physical Therapists' website as a resource for finding physical therapists who have completed rigorous fellowship training aligned with these characteristics.

Mental Healthcare Professionals

Research shows that chronic low-back pain, especially when accompanied by stress, anxiety, or depression, responds well to the mind-based treatment approaches discussed in chapter 14. The healthcare professionals most likely to offer these approaches include psychologists, psychiatrists (medical physicians who specialize in mental health), social workers, and mental health therapists/counselors. According to pain psychologist Dr. Kerns, whom you met in prior chapters, research shows that several mental health professionals, including psychologists, social workers, and mental health counselors, can deliver effective psychologically based care. What matters is whether they have the expertise and training to treat patients with chronic pain. In addition to the traditional talk therapy used to address stress, anxiety, and depression, pain psychologists and some social workers are also trained in CBT and behavioral therapies. This training allows them to specifically focus on helping people who are experiencing the emotions and feelings frequently experienced by those living with chronic pain, including fear avoidance and ONTs.

Training and credentials:

Most mental healthcare professionals hold a graduate-level education and must be licensed by the state to practice. Psychologists have a PhD or PsyD, while psychiatrists have an MD with specialty training in mental health. Some advanced practice nurses also specialize in mental health. All are trained to perform psychological assessments, identify mental health conditions, and provide psychotherapy/counseling. Most licensed clinical social workers hold at least a master's degree and can help individuals advocate for themselves within their communities and provide mental health support. Mental health therapists or counselors usually have master's-level training and often have special areas of focus, such as depression, anxiety, or alcohol and drug addiction/abuse.

The American Psychological Association (APA) is developing a micro-credential for pain that will require specific training for professionals. However, as of the writing of this book, it is not yet available. The APA is also working with states to implement continuing education for existing licensed providers, including psychologists, social workers, master's-level mental health counselors, and even psychology technicians. Credentials specifically for mental health approaches to pain management do not yet exist.

Treatment approaches:

Talk therapy, cognitive behavioral therapy, and behavioral therapy. Psychiatrists can also prescribe medication. Advanced practice nurses and physician assistants can also prescribe medication, though their rules for prescribing controlled substances vary by state.

Finding the right person:

Identifying the right mental healthcare professional can be challenging due to the high demand and limited supply. Dr. Kerns recommends that, if you are working with another healthcare professional to manage your low back pain, ask for a recommendation or referral to a mental health professional they partner with, either in the community or maybe even within their practice. If you have third-party coverage that includes pain psychology, ask your health insurance company for a list of approved mental healthcare professionals specializing in pain management.

The magazine *Psychology Today* publishes a list of psychologists searchable by zip code. However, Dr. Kerns advises that if you go this route, do so knowing you can't assume anything about quality or credentials from these lists.

Costs:

Although better outcomes are not associated with any specific credential, some third-party payers may limit coverage to mental health care delivered by psychologists or social workers. These payment policies vary by health insurance company and by state. Further, many mental healthcare professionals who specialize in helping people living with pain don't accept any insurance.

Other considerations:

Based on conversations with Dr. Kerns:

- While the number of visits with a mental healthcare professional will vary depending on your needs as an individual, around ten visits is common.
- Regardless of the credentials of the mental healthcare professional you see, expect to receive a comprehensive assessment of your mental health, goal setting based on your individual needs, and shared decision-making about what course of treatment is best for you.

- Gain insight into whether a mental healthcare professional is right for you by requesting a brief phone conversation or initial consultation with any psychologist or social worker that you are considering. Questions to ask include: "Do you have expertise in treating patients with low back pain?" "What is your background and training?" "What should I expect if I were to see you regarding assessment and developing treatment goals?" "How long is the typical course of therapy?" "What treatment approach or approaches do you take?"

- If you are considering CBT-based group therapy, you will want to consider a range of factors. Individual therapy sessions offer privacy, one-on-one attention, and a personalized approach. Group sessions offer the potential benefits of support and encouragement from others, as well as a sense of shared experiences that can help alleviate feelings of isolation.

- Only a subset of mental healthcare professionals is allowed to diagnose mental health conditions. These include psychiatrists, psychologists, advanced practice nurses, and licensed clinical social workers.

- Two of the most important contributors to the success of mental health treatment approaches are whether you like and trust your mental healthcare professional and if you believe that the recommended treatment approaches will be helpful to you.

Note: Some people do not believe that a mental healthcare professional is the right fit for them. If this is true for you, but you are experiencing stress, anxiety, or depression, discuss this with your clinician, regardless of their background and training. If a direct conversation on this issue feels uncomfortable to you, consider asking more indirect questions. Examples include: "How would you manage somebody who is experiencing anxiety or depression?" or "What is your general approach to managing somebody who has a lot of back pain and maybe is a little stressed out about it?"

Key Takeaways

- The type of healthcare professional you choose to help you on your healing journey can have a big influence on the trajectory of your low back pain outcomes.
- There are several things you should expect from any health-care professional that you consult. These include respect for you as a person, their willingness to work with you as an active partner in managing your low back pain, and a focus on guideline-recommended treatment approaches.
- Chiropractors are trained to diagnose, manage, and treat low back pain using treatment approaches such as spinal manipulation.
- Physical therapists are trained to manage and treat low back pain using treatment approaches such as super-vised exercise and mobilization.
- Mental healthcare professionals, including psychol-ogists, social workers, and counselors, can provide support for patients living with chronic low back pain, especially those who are also experiencing stress, anxiety, or depression.

chapter 19

Medical Professionals

In chapter 4, you learned that adhering to the strictly biomedical model may not be the best way to start when it comes to managing low back pain. However, as you will learn in this chapter, medical physicians and other medical professionals—primary care physicians (family practice, general internist, osteopathic physicians), physician assistants and advanced practice nurses, nonsurgical spine specialists, and spine surgeons—can play an essential role.

As is true for all clinicians treating low back pain, your medical professional should take a detailed history, conduct a physical examination, and listen carefully to you as you describe your low back pain and how it is impacting your life. They should ask good questions and be prepared to answer any questions you might have. They should focus on guideline-recommended care for low back pain. Finally, they should engage with you in shared decision-making and ensure you understand the benefits and risks of all your pain management options.

Primary Care Physicians

Primary care physicians have a doctorate in medicine (MD) or osteopathy (DO) and work as family practice physicians, general internists, or pediatricians. Most people turn to one of these healthcare professionals first for most or all of their healthcare needs. The US medical system is designed that way because primary care physicians are well trained to diagnose and manage a broad range of healthcare conditions. They can serve as gatekeepers to advanced diagnostic testing and specialty care. Having one person responsible for coordinating your care is efficient and effective. This coordination is especially critical for people with multiple conditions, such as diabetes, hypertension, gastrointestinal issues, or heart disease.

About half of patients seeking care for low back pain start with a primary care physician. There are several good reasons to do so. First, many people already have a relationship with a primary care physician. Second, individuals with low back pain often have other health conditions that respond well to medical management, creating the allure of a "one-stop" approach to

care. Third, health insurance plans are likely to pay for primary care visits. Finally, primary care physicians are available in many communities.

However, primary care practitioners face several challenges when treating low back pain. First, as you have already learned, the biomedical model taught in medical school does not offer a cure or even a universally safe and effective approach. Second, patients often have multiple reasons for their primary care visit. The limited time of a typical PCP visit may not be long enough to effectively address your low back pain and effectively manage these other health conditions, determine what treatments might work best for you, talk with you about all the potential benefits and side effects, engage with you in shared decision-making about next steps, and write everything down in the electronic health record. Third, most primary care physicians lack training in Whole Health approaches and guideline-recommended treatments, such as acupuncture and manual therapies.

Treatment approaches:

Prescription medications, patient education, and referrals for diagnostic tests, medical specialty care, physical therapy, or chiropractic care.

Training and credentials:

Primary care physicians must complete a four-year undergraduate degree program, four years of medical school (earning an MD or DO degree), and at least three years of residency training, typically in family medicine or internal medicine. They are also required to pass the United States Medical Licensing Examination and obtain licensure in the state(s) in which they practice. Dr. Krebs recommends that you look for a physician with current specialty board certification, as this certification requires regular testing of updated medical knowledge. You can look up your medical physician on the American Board of Medical Specialties website. Locate the For Patients tab and enter your physician's last name and the state in which they practice in the search engine.

Finding the right person:

Pick a primary care physician who has a specific interest and expertise in treating low back pain. You want someone who knows and follows low back pain guidelines. Someone who does not order early imaging and who has a broad range of referral sources, including chiropractors, acupuncturists, physical therapists, and medical specialists. Someone who takes a patient-centered perspective and is interested in working with you on your Whole Health approach to healing over the long run, rather than short-term symptom management.

Costs:

The cost of seeing a primary care physician varies widely by location, the health system in which they work, and the type of health insurance you use. However, in general, health insurance plans tend to cover most, if not all, of the cost of seeing a primary care physicians.

Other considerations:

When seeking a medical physician to help with your low back pain, you may want to consider a doctor of osteopathic Medicine (DO). DOs attend medical schools similar to those that train medical physicians, and most participate in the same residency programs as their medical physician colleagues. However, early in its history, osteopathy emphasized the role of the spine, nerves, and other components of the musculoskeletal system in addressing disease. As a result, although doctors of osteopathic medicine provide prescription medications and other biomedical treatments, some also take a more Whole Health approach to patient care. For example, some DOs regularly practice osteopathic manual medicine, which includes manual therapies and spinal manipulation.

Nonsurgical Spine Specialists

Nonsurgical spine specialists include physiatrists, pain management specialists, interventional radiologists, and interventional anesthesiologists. These healthcare professionals can help you address red flag symptoms and treatment-resistant chronic low back pain that interferes with your ability to live your life fully.

Treatment approaches:

The approaches used by nonsurgical pain specialists vary by individual physician and the health system in which they work. However, interventional radiologists and anesthesiologists tend to primarily focus on administering interventional procedures. Pain management specialists are most likely to offer interventional procedures and medication management. Physiatrists, sometimes called physical medicine and rehabilitation physicians, take a nonsurgical biomedical approach to pain management and rehabilitation, with a specific focus on improving physical functioning. In addition to interventional procedures, they are the nonsurgical specialists most likely to offer patient education and advice, medication management, and often functional rehabilitation exercises. Some nonsurgical spine specialists also offer acupuncture and, especially if they are DOs, manual therapies.

Training and credentials:

All physicians begin with the same foundational training. Nonsurgical spine specialists must complete a four-year undergraduate degree program, followed by four years of medical school (earning either an MD or a DO degree). After medical school, they complete four years of residency training specifically in their field of study, be it physical medicine and rehabilitation, anesthesiology, pain management, or radiology. In addition, they must complete one to two additional years in a fellowship program learning to administer interventional procedures and other pain management approaches.

Finding the right person:

Sometimes, the purpose of seeing a nonsurgical spine specialist is because you and your medical physician have determined that an interventional procedure is right for you. If so, the person you want to see is the one most experienced in delivering that specific procedure. However, if you are looking for a longer-term partner to help you manage your low back pain, the best place to start may be with a physiatrist. They are most likely to have expertise in treating a broad range of patients with low back pain and often focus on guideline-recommended treatment approaches before turning to prescription medications or interventional procedures.

Here is some advice from Dr. Eubanks on finding the right physiatrist:

- Look for someone who spends more time seeing patients outside the procedure clinic than doing interventional procedures.
- The right physiatrist can be a facilitator who connects patients with trusted chiropractors, physical therapists, or surgeons when necessary.
- They should begin any conversation you have by talking about self-care options and noninvasive, guideline-recommended treatments, including the things that you have already tried.
- Be sure to ask about the likelihood of success and potential risks of any interventional procedure recommended.

- Look for someone who takes your whole body into account and whose primary focus is on your functional outcomes, not on your pain.
- Physiatrists often work as part of interdisciplinary teams that may include physical therapists and pain psychologists. As a result, they may be able to help you coordinate your care if you need to work with multiple healthcare professionals on your care team.

Spine Surgeons

After reading chapter 16 on surgical procedures, you have already learned that surgery is rarely the answer for low back pain. In the process, you also learned quite a bit about spine surgeons. Here are a few more things to keep in mind.

Most spine surgeons are either orthopedic (sometimes also spelled orthopaedic, mostly by academic institutions) surgeons or neurosurgeons. Historically, orthopedic surgeons specialized in the musculoskeletal system, including bones, joints, muscles, and ligaments. In contrast, neurosurgeons focused more on the nervous system, which includes the brain, spinal cord, and nerves. However, when it comes to spine surgeons who specialize in caring for most patients with low back pain, that distinction rarely exists today. In fact, some spine fellowships today are integrated across neurosurgery and orthopedics, and many spine surgeons have had mixed training.

Treatment approaches:

Primarily surgical procedures, with some surgeons also offering interventional procedures, as well as education and advice on nonsurgical treatment options.

Training and credentials:

Spine surgeons complete a four-year undergraduate degree program, followed by four years of medical school (earning either an MD or a DO degree). They must then complete a residency program in either orthopedic surgery (usually five years) or neurosurgery (usually seven years). In general, orthopedic spine surgeons will complete a one-year spine surgery fellowship after residency. Some neurosurgeons may not, since they were exposed to more spine pathology during their residency.

Finding the right person:

As my Duke colleague Dr. Oren Gottfired once told me, "You can't undo back surgery." Thus, you want a spine surgeon who is experienced in the surgical technique that is right for you and has the characteristics I have already discussed for all healthcare professionals. These factors include listening to your concerns, answering your questions, involving you in shared decision-making, and ensuring you are fully informed about the risks and benefits. Here are a few other things to keep in mind:

- The right spine surgeon should feel confident in their ability to help with the specific symptoms you are experiencing. They should have a clear understanding of your needs and be able to articulate how the surgery will address those needs.

- The surgeon should be willing to discuss the number of similar surgeries they have performed within the past year and their level of expertise with the recommended procedure.

- The surgeon should explain your anticipated recovery process in detail, based on you as an individual. They should take your lifestyle and expectations into account. For example, if you are a competitive golfer, the surgeon should understand what recovery means to you and how your recovery timeline may differ from that of someone who leads a less active lifestyle.

- Do your homework when it comes to the surgeon's reputation. Reading online reviews is a good place to start. Dr. Gottfried also recommends asking the nurses and clinical staff during your initial consultation about the surgeon's average outcomes. They are the ones who see how patients are doing when they return for their postoperative visits a few weeks later.

- Dr. Minchew recommends that you ask in advance about the surgeon's level of involvement with your case after the operation is completed. Ask about the timing of postoperative visits and whom you will see during them.

- You will need to figure out for yourself what the right balance is between the surgeon's bedside manner and the odds of achieving the best outcomes possible. Ideally, you want someone who is both compassionate and technically excellent. That mix can be hard to find. You may lean toward technical excellence. However, bedside manner also matters from the perspective of making sure your questions get answered and that you are involved in shared decision-making regarding whether surgery is right for you.

- The right spine surgeon should be open to discussing alternative treatments and making decisions collaboratively with you. You should never feel pressured into surgery.

- The surgeon should be able to provide specific data on complication rates and other objective measures of success based on that specific surgical technique for people who are similar to you.

- Dr. Minchew recommends looking for a surgeon who takes extra care in learning everything about you and your low back pain before surgery. "If they take that much care before getting into the operating room," he says, "that's a good sign that they're going to take that same kind of care inside the operating room."

Costs:

Spine surgery for low back pain can cost anywhere from about $12,000 for a simple procedure to more than $150,000 for complex cases. While most insurance plans cover the costs of approved surgical procedures, significant co-pays may be required. Once again, be sure to check with your insurance company about your financial risk before undergoing spine surgery.

Physician Assistants and Advanced Practice Nurses

Physician assistants (PAs) and nurse practitioners (NPs or APNs) are trained and licensed to treat many common patient health problems. These clinicians are sometimes combined into a category called advanced practice providers (APPs), but they are distinct professions with different training programs. Physician assistants must complete a master's degree from an accredited program, pass the national Physician Assistant National Certifying Examination, and obtain licensure in the state where they will practice. Nurse practitioners must first receive a bachelor of science in nursing, followed by either a master of science in nursing (NP) or doctor of nursing practice (DNP) degree. APPs are required to pass a comprehensive licensing examination sponsored by the appropriate accrediting organization and be licensed by the state(s) in which they practice.

You are very likely to encounter an APP at your medical physician's office, regardless of whether that office is focused on primary care, specialty care, or surgery. APPs are similar to other medical professionals in that they can specialize in many areas. To gain the expertise needed, APPs typically undergo postgraduate fellowship training and earn advanced certifications in their area of interest.

Finding the right APP is more dependent on their specialty area of focus than on their credentials. If your APP's role is that of a primary care clinician, consider the characteristics I listed for primary care physicians. If your APP works closely with either a physiatrist or surgeon, look there for guidance instead.

Key Takeaways

- Regardless of the initials after your medical professional's name, they should take a detailed history and physical examination, listen carefully to you as you describe your low back pain and how it is impacting your life, and talk with you about the benefits and risks of any recommended treatment approaches.
- Primary care physicians often serve as the first point of contact for patients with low back pain. They can prescribe medications, coordinate care, make referrals to specialists, and manage other health conditions that may coexist with low back pain.
- Advanced practice nurses and physician assistants may serve in either a primary care or specialty care role.
- Nonsurgical spine specialists, such as physiatrists and pain management specialists, can help when low back pain does not respond to self-care or guideline-recommended treatments or when red flag symptoms are present.
- Remember, you can't undo surgery. Your surgeon's technical expertise and approach to helping patients matter more than their specialty as an orthopedic surgeon or a neurosurgeon.

chapter 20

Other Professionals Who Can Help with Your Low Back Pain

If you are struggling to incorporate the Whole Health model into your life or feel overwhelmed when thinking about where to start, consider seeking help from an acupuncturist, a massage therapist, a health coach, yoga instructor, or personal trainer. Keep in mind that these trained professionals are unlikely to be experts in low back pain or, except for acupuncturists, trained to diagnose its causes. What they can do is provide active overall wellness support throughout your low back pain journey.

Health Coaches

In chapter 7, you learned about the importance of self-management, motivation, and resilience in managing low back pain. Sometimes channeling those parts of yourself is straightforward, and at other times, it isn't all that easy. If you're struggling to develop and implement your Take Your Back Back Action Plan, a health coach who routinely works with those experiencing low back pain may be able to help.

Treatment approaches:

Whole Health, self-empowerment, resilience, and motivation.

Training and credentials:

Check that any health coach you consider has been trained by a reputable institution and is credentialed by the National Board for Health and Wellness Coaching (NBHWC) in collaboration with the National Board of Medical Examiners. You will also want someone who has experience working with people who have low back pain. Health coaches support clients in making sustainable lifestyle changes, complementing, but not replacing, clinical care.

Cost:

The cost of a health coach varies from about $50 per hour to more than $500 per hour. Many health coaches offer packages with discounted rates for multiple sessions. Some insurance plans cover wellness coaching. Because this offering is not widely available, check with your insurance company. You may also be able to use your flexible spending account or health savings account to cover the cost of health coaching.

Finding the right person:

Health and wellness coaching is a broad profession that is not as well regulated as other health professions. Anyone can advertise themselves as a health coach, with little to no certification. You can verify a coach's credentials through the NBHWC's official directory, helping you distinguish trained professionals from unregulated practitioners.

Other considerations:

Here are some insights on finding a health coach from conversations with Duke University health coach Anna Batsakes:

- A first session with a health coach can last one to two hours, while follow-up sessions tend to be thirty to forty-five minutes in length.
- Pick someone you like talking with, who listens carefully to what you have to say and takes into consideration where you are on your health journey. Health coaching involves you as an active partner in discovering and developing your health and wellness goals and implementing a sustainable action plan.
- Make sure your health coach is familiar with the Personal Health Inventory or use a similar tool to help you identify your "why," and works with you to develop an individualized coaching plan based on your specific health goals.
- Ask how they are going to help you hold yourself accountable. A skilled coach will help you maintain focus and momentum while allowing room for real life. They will encourage self-reflection,

helping you learn from both successes and challenges, which in turn will help you build confidence and self-trust.

Strength and Conditioning Coaches and Personal Trainers

If you find yourself struggling to develop and/or implement the movement or exercise component of your Take Your Back Back Action Plan, a personal trainer or strength and conditioning coach might be the solution for you. The goal of these coaches is to help you develop an exercise program tailored to your needs, teach you proper exercise technique, and encourage you to stay motivated and continue your program over the long term. While there is some overlap in the tasks performed by each of these professions, personal trainers typically work with a diverse range of fitness levels. Strength and conditioning coaches often focus more on the science of exercise, working with clients interested in developing strength and endurance. Many have a special interest in working with athletes.

Treatment approaches:

Exercise and, sometimes, Whole Health approaches such as nutrition and overall wellness advice.

Training and credentials:

There are no specific educational requirements for either personal trainers or strength and conditioning coaches. However, certification is a requirement for employment at most gyms and other locations where they most often work. The National Commission for Certifying Agencies and the American National Standards Institute both certify organizations that credential these professionals. Certification generally includes an examination and regular continuing education.

Finding the right person:

Ask friends and colleagues for recommendations in your community. Look for a personal trainer or strength and conditioning coach who is certified by an organization that is credentialed by one of the organizations I named above. Ask about your coach's experience working with people like you who have low back pain. Choose someone who can meet you where you are and help you create a personalized exercise plan. This plan should include adapting specific exercises to your abilities and needs when necessary.

Cost:

Individualized training ranges from about $50 to more than $500 per hour, while group sessions can be considerably less expensive. Similar to health coaches, many strength and conditioning coaches and personal trainers offer discounted packages for multiple sessions. Some insurance plans cover the cost of gym memberships or fitness classes. They are less likely to cover the cost of one-on-one training, but check with your insurance company to see if they will cover this expense if a qualified healthcare professional prescribes exercise for your low back pain. You may also be able to use your flexible spending account or health savings account to pay for these services. Even then you will likely need a licensed healthcare professional to write a Letter of Medical Necessity stating that exercise training is required to treat your low back pain.

Yoga Instructors and Yoga Therapists

The goal of yoga instructors and therapists is to help you develop a yoga practice that is right for you, teach you how to breathe and do the poses correctly, and help you stay motivated to practice regularly.

Treatment approaches:

Breathing, exercise, and mindfulness.

Training and credentials:

While there is considerable overlap in work and intent, there are differences in training and client focus between yoga instructors and yoga therapists. Most yoga instructors lead classes designed to promote overall health and well-being. Yoga instructors are required to undergo at least two hundred hours of training in a registered yoga school and then register with the Yoga Alliance to become a Registered Yoga Teacher (RYT-200). More advanced training is also available.

Yoga therapists are more likely to offer one-on-one yoga coaching focused on addressing a specific health condition, such as low back pain. Yoga therapists must complete the same two-hundred-hour training program as yoga instructors, receive an additional eight hundred hours of training at an accredited yoga therapy school, and pass an examination required by the International Association of Yoga Therapists to become a certified yoga therapist (C-IAYT). Regular continuing education is necessary for RYT-certified yoga instructors and therapists.

Finding the right person:

Contact nearby yoga studios, gyms, or YMCAs and ask the owner or manager to recommend a yoga teacher or classes specifically designed for clients with low back pain. An important follow-up question is why they recommend that person or class. Look for yoga teachers who are affiliated with medical programs, chiropractic clinics, physical therapy clinics, and hospitals. Visit the Yoga Alliance website and search their directory for local yoga instructors.

Costs:

The cost of yoga classes or working with a yoga therapist varies widely—many gyms offer free yoga classes with a $50–$60 monthly membership. Yoga studios tend to focus only on yoga but may charge twice that amount or more per month, with the cost of seeing a yoga therapist even higher.

Generally, yoga is not covered by health insurance; however, some insurance plans may cover the cost of gym memberships that offer yoga classes. As with exercise coaches, you may be able to use your flexible spending account or health savings account to pay for yoga, but, once again, you will need a licensed healthcare professional to write a Letter of Medical Necessity stating that yoga is required to treat your low back pain.

Other considerations:

Here are some things to keep in mind when choosing a yoga instructor or therapist, based on conversations with Tanya Witman, LAC, LMT, MA, RYT-200, yoga instructor in Tucson, Arizona:

- Many yoga instructors and therapists are cross-trained in other healthcare professions, such as mental health counseling, acupuncture, physical therapy, and chiropractic. You may want to consider finding someone with dual credentials, especially when you are just beginning to figure out what yoga practice works best for you and your low back.
- Find someone who has been teaching yoga for at least two years. It takes time to hone your skills as a yoga teacher and learn what works best for clients living with low back pain.
- Ask the yoga instructor directly how much experience they have with clients living with low back pain and how they will work with you to modify any poses that might lead to pain or discomfort. Some yoga teachers have also have certifications specifically focused on working with clients living with low back pain. Consider a one-on-one session before taking a group class, or look for a series of classes offered either locally or online that are specifically geared toward patients with low back pain.

Massage Therapists

Massage therapists provide hands-on manual therapies to the muscles, tendons, and ligaments of the body. Their goal is to promote relaxation, improve circulation, relieve pain, and enhance overall well-being.

Treatment approaches:

Massage.

Training and credentials:

The vast majority of states require licensure for massage therapists, which typically involves graduating from an accredited educational program with five hundred to one thousand hours of training, passing the Massage and Bodywork Licensing Examination, and meeting continuing education requirements. States with less stringent requirements include California, where certification is optional; Vermont, where registration is required, but certification or licensure is not; and Kansas, Minnesota, and Wyoming, where massage is not regulated. Licensed massage therapists should possess a fundamental understanding of anatomy and the human body's functioning. However, they are not trained or licensed to diagnose or manage health conditions, including low back pain.

Finding the right person:

Ask friends and colleagues for recommendations in your community. Additionally, check whether a massage therapist is practicing at your local health system, hospital, or medical/chiropractic clinic. You want a massage therapist who has a good working understanding of spine anatomy and physiology, as well as experience working with clients living with low back pain. Look for someone who is a good match for how you prefer to be touched. Some people prefer a gentle touch, while others enjoy a more firm approach. Both types of massage can be effective for low back pain, so it ultimately comes down to your personal preferences.

Consider contacting the massage therapist before scheduling an appointment to discuss their approach to treating clients with low back pain and address any other questions you may have. Expect the massage therapist to ask you questions as well. Examples include: "What has your experience been with massage previously?" "Are there things about that massage that you found helpful or did not find helpful?" If you're new to massages, the therapist may ask what you hope to achieve from it or if any aspects of massage make you feel uncomfortable.

Costs:

The cost of seeing a massage therapist varies based on the length of the session, the environment in which the massage therapist practices (massage at medical clinics is often more expensive than in private practice or health spas), and what the local market will bear. Typically, the cost of a one-hour massage ranges from $75 to $150. You may also be able to use your flexible spending account or health savings account to see a massage therapist.

Other considerations:

- Most massages last between 30 and 90 minutes.
- On your first visit, the massage therapist should ask you to complete a patient history form and discuss your low back pain and any other health issues you are either experiencing now or have experienced in the past.
- Before your massage, don't be afraid to tell the therapist about your past massage experiences if you have them, such as "the last massage therapist I saw was so gentle, it didn't really help

with my low back pain," or "they used so much pressure I felt worse afterward." You should also feel comfortable giving the massage therapist feedback during the massage itself, such as "that's a little too much pressure," or "I feel like you're not really getting deep enough into where I'm in pain."

- If you tried massage and didn't like it, don't automatically assume that massage is not right for you. If you feel uncomfortable about massages in general, or if you dislike being touched by people you do not know well, massage may not be the best fit. However, if there were aspects of your last massage that worked for you and others that didn't, think specifically about what didn't work. Examples might include too much pressure, not enough pressure, the therapist talking all the way through the massage, or the therapist not explaining what they were doing or why. These are things to discuss with the massage therapist during that initial phone call. You are likely to find someone who is a better match for your preferences and needs.

Acupuncturists

While some medical physicians, chiropractors, and physical therapists provide acupuncture or dry needling, this section is focused specifically on acupuncturists. Depending on the state in which they are credentialed and the academic program from which they graduated, acupuncturists may be referred to as doctors of Oriental medicine, licensed acupuncturists, registered acupuncturists, or acupuncture physicians. For simplicity's sake, I will use the term acupuncturist here. Acupuncturists take a Whole Health or integrative approach to caring for patients with a wide range of health-related conditions. These include low back pain itself but also many Back Factors, like stress, fatigue, and anxiety.

Treatment approaches:

Acupuncture and sometimes education, overall wellness advice, herbal medicine, and other traditional Chinese medicine treatments.

Training and credentials:

Acupuncturists must complete a four-year master's-level program at an accredited academic institution, in addition to at least sixty hours of undergraduate training. In most states, acupuncturists must also pass a mandatory exam administered by the National Certification Commission for Acupuncture and Oriental Medicine and meet individual state licensing requirements to become a licensed acupuncturist (LAC) or a national board-certified acupuncturist (NBCA). Doctors of acupuncture (DAC) undergo an additional two years of postgraduate training.

Finding the right person:

Ask friends and colleagues for recommendations in your community. Additionally, check whether there is an acupuncturist practicing in your local health system, hospital, or medical/chiropractic clinic. Another option is to visit the National Certification Commission for Acupuncture and Oriental Medicine website and search their database of board-certified acupuncturists. You can also check whether your state has a board of acupuncture with a searchable database of licensed acupuncturists in your area.

Costs:

The cost of seeing an acupuncturist varies widely, but it typically ranges from $100 to $200 for the initial visit and $50 to $100 for subsequent follow-up visits. While this varies significantly based on one's underlying condition, six to eight visits should give you a pretty good idea of whether acupuncture is working for you. Some insurance plans cover visits to an acupuncturist or doctor of Oriental medicine, but this varies widely, so it is essential to check before making an appointment. Not all trained professionals who provide acupuncture accept insurance, and some insurance plans cover acupuncture only if specific trained professionals offer it. Ironically, those trained professionals are more likely to be medical professionals than acupuncturists. You may be able to use your flexible spending account or health savings account to cover the cost of visits with either an acupuncturist or a doctor of Oriental medicine.

Other considerations:

- Acupuncturists inherently take a Whole Health approach to healing, one that is rooted in ancient healing traditions. As a result, your acupuncturist may use methods to diagnose your condition that are unfamiliar, such as evaluating your pulses or looking at your tongue. Ask them to clearly explain any diagnostic tests, diagnoses, and the details of the recommended treatment plan.
- They should use disposable needles.
- It is normal to experience a range of sensations in the areas where needles are inserted. Your acupuncturist should advise you to let them know if you start to feel uncomfortable in any way.
- Acupuncture needles are usually left in for twenty to thirty minutes after insertion. If the acupuncturist leaves you alone to rest during that time, they should check in after a few minutes to ensure that you are still comfortable and address any questions you may have. This is especially important on your first visit.

Choose a Qualified Healthcare Professional

Choosing whether to see a healthcare professional and then selecting that person is among the most impactful decisions you will make when managing your low back pain. Given your many choices, this decision may seem complicated.

Here are three key action steps that can make it easier:

1. Match your Back Factors to the best treatment approach, as you did at the end of part 2.
2. Consider practicalities like availability, cost, and personal preferences.
3. Match your best treatment approach to the right healthcare professional, using figure 10.

Don't be surprised if your treatment approaches lead you to more than one healthcare professional. A team approach is often best, especially for chronic low back pain.

List your healthcare professional options here.

Note that an asterisk after a health profession in figure 10 indicates that only some clinicians within that profession offer the treatment approach indicated.

Healthcare professional #1 ______________________

Healthcare professional #2 ______________________

Healthcare professional #3 ______________________

Healthcare professional #4 ______________________

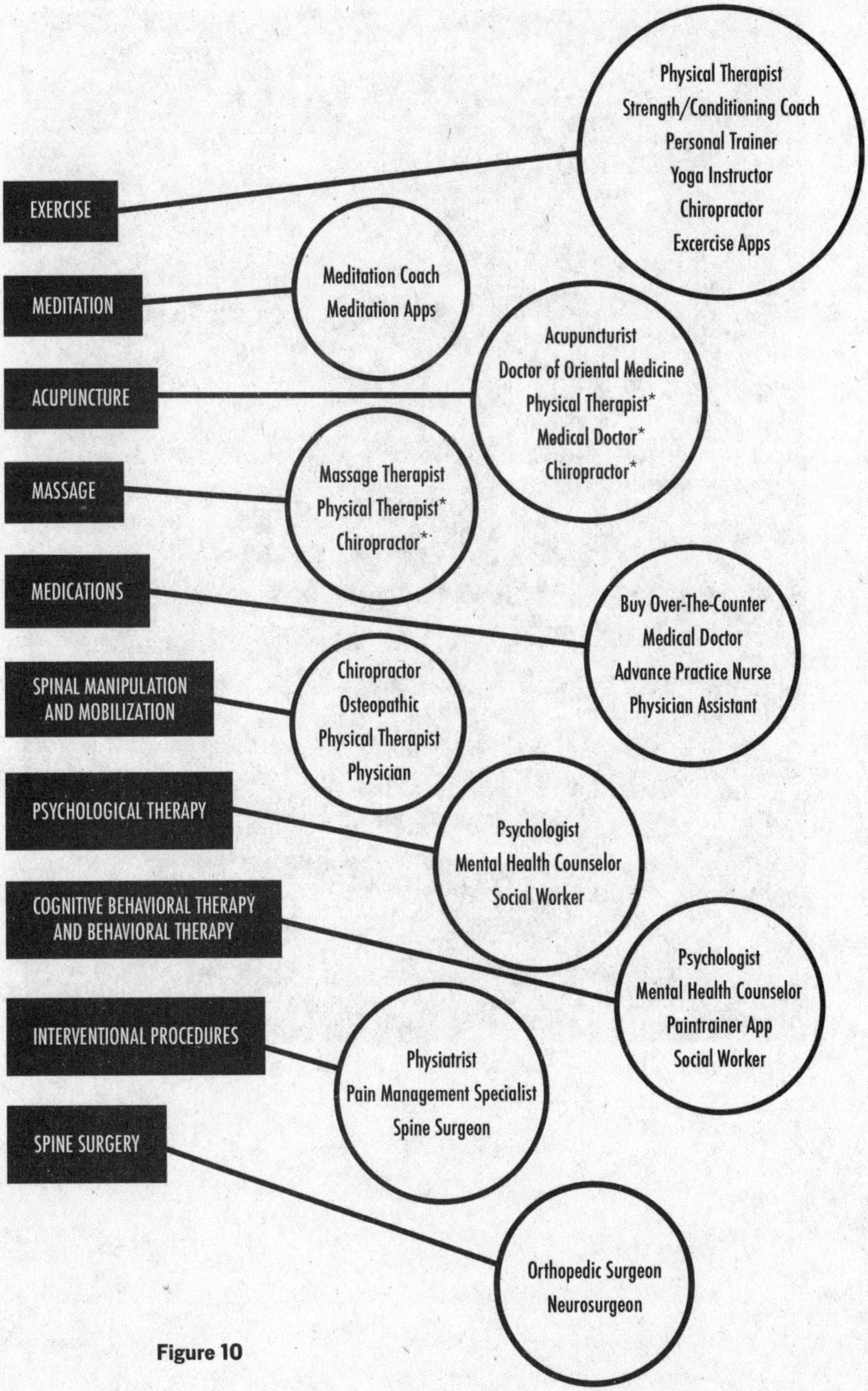
EXERCISE
Physical Therapist
Strength/Conditioning Coach
Personal Trainer
Yoga Instructor
Chiropractor
Excercise Apps
MEDITATION
Meditation Coach
Meditation Apps
ACUPUNCTURE
Acupuncturist
Doctor of Oriental Medicine
Physical Therapist*
Medical Doctor*
Chiropractor*
MASSAGE
Massage Therapist
Physical Therapist*
Chiropractor*
MEDICATIONS
Buy Over-The-Counter
Medical Doctor
Advance Practice Nurse
Physician Assistant
SPINAL MANIPULATION AND MOBILIZATION
Chiropractor
Osteopathic
Physical Therapist
Physician
PSYCHOLOGICAL THERAPY
Psychologist
Mental Health Counselor
Social Worker
COGNITIVE BEHAVIORAL THERAPY AND BEHAVIORAL THERAPY
Psychologist
Mental Health Counselor
Paintrainer App
Social Worker
INTERVENTIONAL PROCEDURES
Physiatrist
Pain Management Specialist
Spine Surgeon
SPINE SURGERY
Orthopedic Surgeon
Neurosurgeon

Figure 10

Key Takeaways

- Many trained professionals can assist you in taking a Whole Health approach to managing your low back pain, including health coaches, yoga instructors, strength and conditioning coaches, massage therapists, and acupuncturists.
- These trained professionals can provide Whole Health support during your low back pain journey but are not experts in diagnosing or managing low back pain.
- Finding the right trained professional to help with your Whole Health journey can be challenging. Ask your health-care professionals, family, friends, and colleagues for recommendations or turn to professional and accrediting organizations for searchable lists of options in your area.
- Always choose trained professionals who have certifications from reputable institutions and have experience working with individuals with low back pain.
- Your insurance plan is less likely to cover the costs of seeing the trained professionals described in this chapter, so it is important to understand the costs up front.

chapter 21

Advocate for Yourself

I wish this chapter was not needed. I wish that every person facing low back pain could easily get the right care at the right time, at an affordable cost. Unfortunately, that is not happening consistently enough, at least in the United States. As David Elton, DC, cofounder of Arete Healthcare and CEO of Arete Networks told me, "The average consumer must navigate a health system full of misinformation and poorly aligned incentives." Despite new research and guideline development over the past decade, there is a significant gap between established best practices for low back pain and actual clinical practice. Many of the reasons for this gap stem from the fact that change is difficult within entrenched healthcare delivery systems.

Using the power of your own voice can help you overcome these challenges. Thus, the last step before you begin developing your Take Your Back Back Action Plan is to learn how to advocate for yourself.

Advocating for Yourself with Healthcare Professionals

I introduced you to the Spine Squad in chapter 4, when discussing how complex it can be to determine the causes of low back pain. The Spine Squad also talked about how they advocated for themselves when working with healthcare professionals. One of them said, "I track everything—my pain levels, what triggers them—so doctors can't dismiss me." If you also sometimes feel dismissed by your healthcare professional, here are some suggestions to help you get the most out of your visit.

- Write your questions down in advance in the order of their importance and walk into the medical physician's office with your list in hand.
- Bring a friend or family member with you to help you stay focused on your needs. That person may also be able to provide additional

context on how low back pain is impacting not just your life but also the lives of the people around you.

- Be prepared to ask a question multiple times if you don't get an answer the first time. Don't allow a clinician to brush you off. Low back pain is complex. It's important to ask questions if you don't understand what has been said or need additional clarification. Keep asking questions until you get answers that make sense to you.

- Keep the healthcare professional focused on the reason for your visit, even if they want to discuss other health issues. Remember Dr. Krebs, whom you first met in earlier chapters? She recommends a two-step approach: acknowledge and refocus. If your clinician begins discussing your high blood pressure or diabetes, pay attention. But don't lose track of the purpose of your visit. If you need to, practice saying things ahead of time, like "I really care about my hypertension or diabetes, but today I am here because of my low back pain. Can we talk about that now? I will make another appointment to talk about my high blood pressure and diabetes on another day."

- Your clinician should listen to what you have to say and take the time to answer your questions. "If your healthcare professional tries to avoid your questions or doesn't give you time to ask those questions, it could be that the person is not a good fit for you," Dr. Krebs says. "But it could also be that they don't have time right then." Ask if you need to make another appointment to finish discussing your low back pain.

- Do your homework before walking into the clinician's office. Know your Back Factors. Tell the clinician that you want to focus on guideline-recommended care. Describe which treatment you believe would be the best fit, and explain why. Feel free to bring a copy of *Take Your Back Back* with you to help with that discussion.

- If your insurance company or flexible spending plan covers treatments like yoga, exercise, or massage, and you need a medical physician's note or prescription, ask for that referral note or prescription. Often, your clinician will be more than happy to help you. If not, ask them to clearly explain why. If that explanation doesn't make sense or is inconsistent with what you know about low back pain treatment guidelines, consider finding another clinician.
- By now, you have a good idea of which treatments are recommended for low back pain. Ask your clinician about manual therapies, mind-based approaches, and exercise. If your clinician is focusing on only one of several treatments that match your Back Factors (e.g., exercise), ask how to access other approaches.
- Remember that starting with early MRIs, corticosteroid injections, prescription medications, and surgery is not the right way to go for most people. If you do specifically ask for those options during your medical physician's visit, you may end up with what you requested, even if it is not the best approach for you at that time.

Advocating for Yourself with Your Insurance Company

The Spine Squad also had a few things to say about their experiences with insurance companies: "The insurance companies are writing the prescriptions, not the doctors, and we, the patients, are stuck suffering." "They tell me to try movement therapy, but my insurance won't pay for it. What am I supposed to do?"

Health insurance plans and policy experts are aware of this issue, and some are working to address the challenges patients face in accessing recommended care for low back pain. America's Health Insurance Plans published a white paper on their website in 2019 that outlined this challenge and offered solutions. The paper called for a whole-person approach to treating low back pain and emphasized the need for broader use of treatments recommended by the ACP. Hopefully, by the time you are reading this book, some of these recommended changes have been implemented. Presuming that is not yet the case, here is a brief recap of several payment issues currently associated with different low back pain treatment options. Keep in mind that this information is "on average." Your situation could be very different.

- You will likely need to pay outright for most of the over-the-counter treatment options described in chapter 11. The same is true for health coaching, personal trainers, yoga, and massage. Insurance may cover gym memberships or group fitness classes, but rarely one-on-one training. However, if a qualified professional prescribes exercise for your low back pain, check with your insurer—coverage may be available. It is worth asking your health plan about this option. Flexible spending or health savings accounts can also help pay for these services.
- The extent to which manual therapies, acupuncture, and behavioral therapies are covered varies a great deal depending on your specific insurance coverage. Often, the co-payments are the same as or more than the cost of the treatment provided, prior authorization is required, or arbitrary limits are set on the number of visits allowed. Generally, insurance covers manual therapies more often than acupuncture or behavioral therapies.
- The majority of health plans cover most or all of the cost to see a primary care physician and often pay much of the cost for prescription medications. They are also likely to pay for corticosteroid injections, radiofrequency ablation, spinal cord stimulators, and spine surgery. However, prior authorization or a failed trial of physical therapy is often required before procedures and surgery.
- Insurance is less likely to pay for prolotherapy, stem cell treatments, or platelet-rich plasma injections.

Okay, enough about the problem. The remainder of this chapter focuses on solutions. You have a lot more power than you may realize when it comes to navigating the health insurance system. That power lies in understanding your total benefits package, understanding the appeals process, educating your employer, and fighting for better access to guideline-recommended care for low back pain. Below are a few action steps you can take to advocate for yourself. In doing so, you may also help some of the 619 million other people on this planet who are currently living with low back pain each year.

As you dive in, realize that this process may be frustrating at times. Your total benefit package is a patchwork of multiple vendors and plans, so following this advice can easily lead to multiple phone calls and emails. However, your persistence will pay off if you discover that the care you need is more available to you than you initially thought.

1. **Make your plan:**

   Review the treatment approaches that best fit with your Back Factors and which healthcare professionals you want on your team. Be clear in your mind about the care you are seeking.

2. **Do your homework:**

   If you do not have health insurance coverage, call the health system or clinic where you hope to seek care and ask to speak with a billing representative to understand the costs associated with the care you need.

3. **Identify financial options:**

   If you cannot afford to pay for the care that you need, talk with your healthcare professional or healthcare delivery system. See what options they have available for self-pay patients with limited incomes.

4. **Understand your insurance:**

   If you do have insurance coverage, review your "evidence of coverage" documents. You should have received a copy of this information the last time you renewed your health insurance, and you can also find it on your health plan's website. Your evidence of coverage document lists which treatments are covered, cost limitations, and the out-of-pocket costs you are responsible for paying directly. It may or may not provide details on existing restrictions regarding which healthcare professionals are authorized to provide those services.

5. **Get help:**
   If you can't locate your evidence of coverage documents or still have questions, call the health insurance company directly using the number on the back of your insurance card. Ask to speak with someone who can answer your coverage questions. You can say something along the lines of "I'm interested in spinal manipulation, massage, or acupuncture to help me manage my low back pain. Can you please tell me whether or not my health insurance includes coverage for any of these?" Write down the name of every person you speak with, as it may be helpful to refer to those conversations later.

6. **Identify your healthcare professional:**
   If necessary, follow up with questions about whether your plan requires you to see specific healthcare professionals, in terms of either licensing and credentials or individual people. They will have a directory of in-network clinicians that allows you to search for options in your area.

7. **Be persistent:**
   If you are told that a specific treatment option or a specific healthcare professional is not one of your covered benefits, don't give up. Ask more questions. Insurance plans often provide discounted access to specific treatment approaches, such as massage, acupuncture, or health coaching. Ensure the person you are speaking with understands that you are not just inquiring about your medical benefits. You also want to make sure you know your entire benefit package. For example, some employee assistance programs provide behavioral health services for

conditions such as depression and anxiety, even though they are not a covered benefit per se. Additionally, your employer may offer value-added benefits, such as gym memberships or health coaching.

8. **Assess all healthcare professional options:**
   It may not cost you any more out of pocket to see a clinician who is not in your health plan network, especially if that clinician is a physical therapist or chiropractor. Often, large co-pays and deductibles mean that patients are already responsible for a significant portion of the cost when seeing these clinicians.

9. **Be even more persistent:**
   The first person you talk to is likely working out of a call center and may not be able to answer all your questions. If that happens, ask if there is someone else you can talk with about coverage issues.

Advocating for Yourself with Your Employer

If you get your health insurance through your employer, talk to your employer's human resources representative if you still have questions or are not satisfied with the answers you got after calling the insurance company directly. Explain your needs and the homework you have done so far regarding review of your evidence of coverage, and repeat the conversation you had with your health insurance plan. Ask for help. "Employee benefits (health insurance provided by an employer) are designed or chosen by your employer," says Doug Metz, DC, former chairman of the URAC Health Standards Committee. "Talking with your human resources representative provides an opportunity to: 1) be sure you fully understand what is or is not covered; (2) obtain advice about how to talk with the insurance company about your specific questions; and (3) advocate for changes in coverage that will help you and others with similar low back pain situations." By educating your employer through your questions and suggestions, you help them identify ways to reduce healthcare costs, retain employees, and provide safe, effective services that research shows can result in fewer days lost from work.

Advocating for Yourself Through the Medical Appeals Process

If your insurance company denies a claim for guideline-recommended care for low back pain, that does not necessarily mean this is the last word on the subject. Every insurance company has an appeals process for denied claims. Few people turn to an appeal when they need it. In 2023, only 1 percent of denied claims were appealed by the patient. Of those appeals, almost half were successful. Many times, the insurance company did not get enough or the correct information from the clinician to approve payment. So, keep going after that first rejection. Here are some things to keep in mind when you do:

- As part of the Affordable Care Act, most insurance plans are required by law to offer patients a process for appealing denied medical claims. The first step in this process is to appeal directly to the insurance company. After the insurance company process is completed, a review by an independent third party is required if the original appeal is denied. Keep in mind that you need to ask for each step. Any denial letters you get from your insurance company are required to include information on how to take the next step in the appeal process.
- The appeals process I am describing generally applies to claims associated with covered benefits rather than treatment approaches that are listed as exclusions. For example, your appeal is likely to be successful if you and your healthcare professional can adequately document why, according to accepted clinical guidelines, you require ten physical therapy visits due to your specific low back pain condition. Your appeal is unlikely

to be successful if your plan does not cover physical therapy at all or doesn't cover physical therapy for your type of low back pain.

- If your original claim is denied, you will receive a letter from the insurance company explaining the reason for the denial, informing you that you have a right to appeal, and providing information on the appeals process. Always appeal.
- If you need additional information about the appeals process, call your insurance company (there should be a phone number in the appeal letter) or look on their website for information on their medical claims appeals process. Detailed information should be readily available. It is essential to follow these instructions. The Patient Advocate Foundation or other similar organizations in your community may be able to help with your appeal if you have questions.
- Request your claims file from the insurance company. Your claims file includes all the documents and other communications that the insurance company is using to process your claim. This will provide information that can help you with your claims appeal. It also shows the insurance company that you are serious about pursuing your appeal. ProPublica has a website that can help you through this process. You will find a link to this website in the resources section at the end of the book.
- Always speak with your healthcare professional first before filing an appeal. You will likely need to provide your medical records to support the claim that the denied care was medically necessary. Your healthcare professional may have additional information that can strengthen your case or discover that they made an error in billing that, when corrected, solves the problem.
- In addition to your medical records, you will be required to write a letter outlining what care was denied and why you need it.
- You can submit your claim by either regular mail or on the insurance company's website. If you choose regular mail, consider sending your

appeal via registered mail so that you can track its arrival. If you submit your claim on the insurance company's website, be sure to upload all your supporting documents.

- If the insurance company denies your appeal, you have the right to an outside review by an independent party. Instructions for initiating this process should be included in the denial letter. Always take that option!

Dr. Vivi-Ann Fischer, former chief clinical officer at Fulcrum Health, recognizes that you may be hesitant to go down the appeals path. However, she recommends considering this option if your claim for guideline-recommended care is denied. "Health plans actually really listen to their members," she says. "Be honest. Explain what you need in your own words. State why you believe the requested care will improve your condition. If you do this, that claim will often be approved. It may be that an error in the system or a lack of sufficient information led to the denial in the first place."

Advocating for Change

Perhaps you found the process of advocating for your needs in the clinician's office or negotiating with your insurance company exciting or motivating. If so, I invite you to join me in another advocacy challenge. That challenge lies in aligning politics and health policy with best practices for managing low back pain at scale, for everyone.

Advocating on your own behalf and for others can feel overwhelming. This work is even more challenging while you are living with chronic back pain. I get that. But before you rule out advocating for change, let me introduce you to Cindy Steinberg, who demonstrates the difference one person can make in the lives of many more.

More than twenty-five years ago, Cindy experienced a serious injury that left her with debilitating thoracic back pain that, in time, progressed to her lower back. "It was absolutely devastating. I had to give up my career. You lose your self-esteem, your whole identity. Along the way, I faced messages that were hard to hear, like you've got to manage this yourself, and there is no magic bullet, and it's messy getting to what's going to help you."

It took Cindy five years to find the right doctor, an osteopathic physician. "'Look,' the doctor said to me. 'I think you have a chronic pain condition where there's no cure.'" He was honest, compassionate, and willing to help her find solutions. "He said, 'I will work with you to find ways to manage the pain to more tolerable levels,'" Cindy says. "For the first time in five years, I felt like I wasn't alone, flailing about, trying and failing treatments. Now I had a partner." Her new doctor had a network of healthcare professionals that he worked with, including a Russian physical therapist who had developed a program of water exercises for musculoskeletal pain and injuries. "The DO sent me to other healthcare professionals and then asked me to come back and report to him on whether the treatment was helping," Cindy says. "I had never had a doctor like that. Before, they would try something, like medication, and if that didn't work, they would say, 'I can't help you.'"

Today, as the director of policy and advocacy for the US Pain Foundation, Cindy is trying to keep people living with chronic pain from feeling as alone as she once did. Part of that work is meeting hundreds of people living with chronic pain, including the more than six hundred people who have participated in the support group that she started twenty-five years ago as a volunteer. However, you are just as likely to find her at a state capitol building or on Capitol Hill advocating for ways to improve pain care through public policy and health systems. A significant part of this is ensuring healthcare providers and people living with pain are educated on the guideline-recommended treatment approaches described in *Take Your Back Back*. In addition to her own advocacy work, she teaches an annual advocacy and pain policy webinar series to help people become more aware of how they can get involved and what they can do, and that their voice matters. You can learn more about Cindy's work and the US Pain Foundation on the US Pain Foundation website.

Key Takeaways

- Access to guideline-recommended care for low back pain remains challenging, even with extensive research and guidelines available to show the way.
- Insurance coverage for effective nondrug treatments like physical therapy, chiropractic care, and acupuncture is often limited or comes with high out-of-pocket costs, despite guideline recommendations.
- Understanding your insurance benefits, evidence of coverage, and the appeals process empowers you to fight for better access to guideline-recommended low back pain care.
- Actively advocating for yourself with clinicians and insurance plans until you receive clear answers and access to the care you need is an important part of self-managing your low back pain.
- Advocating for change at the policy level and within your employer or health system can help improve access to affordable, guideline-concordant care for everyone living with low back pain.

chapter 22

The Take Your Back Back Action Plan

You have learned the basics of low-back pain, including letting go of common myths and identifying your Back Factors. You understand that taking a Whole Health approach to life can help heal low back pain and many other health conditions. You know that self-empowerment, motivation, and resilience are the building blocks to living your best life. You have learned which low back pain treatment approaches are safest and most effective. You know what characteristics to look for when seeking help from a healthcare professional. You can advocate for yourself with both clinicians and insurance companies. Now it is time to put this knowledge to work by following this six-step process to develop and implement your personalized Take Your Back Back Action Plan.

Step 1: Commit to Action

I have already talked about the importance of self-management in addressing low back pain. This means taking ownership of your health, recognizing your strengths, facing your obstacles, and using this information to live the life you want. The first step is to commit to managing your low back pain. You can either sign right here or on a separate sheet of paper. Keep in mind as you make this commitment that success is more about the small commitments you make each day that move you slowly and surely closer to your goals.

I, ____,
commit to taking the actions required each day to heal my low back pain.

Step 2: Pick Your Approach

First, review the Back Factors you identified in chapter 4. List them here.

Back Factor #1 ______________________

Back Factor #2 ______________________

Back Factor #3 ______________________

Back Factor #4 ______________________

Back Factor #5 ______________________

Second, review the treatment approaches you identified at the end of part 2. List them here.

Treatment Approach #1 ______________________

Treatment Approach #2 ______________________

Treatment Approach #3 ______________________

Treatment Approach #4 ______________________

You likely ended up with more than one treatment option. Since you cannot do everything all at once, set priorities based on the following: (1) the Back Factors having the greatest impact on your life; and (2) where there is the most factor overlap. For example, exercise is helpful for three factors: anxiety, arthritis-related pain, and trouble sleeping. If you have any of these Back Factors, I recommend making exercise a priority.

Consider other issues as well, such as what treatments you tried before that either worked or didn't work. Research indicates that treatment approaches that have been effective for a person in the past are likely to be effective again. Another thing to consider is what treatment options are available to you, given your location, lifestyle, and budget.

If the treatment approaches you choose require the help of a healthcare professional, move to step 3. If your treatment approaches are all self-care strategies, skip ahead to step 4.

Step 3: Choose a Qualified Healthcare Professional

If needed, review the healthcare professionals you identified in part 3. List them here.

Healthcare Professional #1 ______________________

Healthcare Professional #2 ______________________

Healthcare Professional #3 ______________________

Healthcare Professional #4 ______________________

If you are working with multiple clinicians to manage your low back pain, make sure they are aware of one another and of all the treatment approaches you are using. If your healthcare professionals work within the same health system, your electronic medical record should do that job for you. If not, ask any clinicians outside the system to send a copy of your medical records to the other healthcare professionals involved in your care.

Step 4: Develop Your Plan

You have the knowledge you need to manage your low back pain. You have identified the Back Factors contributing to your pain and matched them with the right treatment options. You have considered whether self-care or working with a healthcare professional is right for you. Now bring this information together to develop your Action Plan. You can do this independently or ask a healthcare professional for help. Write down your Action Plan. Your plan can start as simple or as detailed as you like.

Begin by looking at how you rated each of the nine domains of well-being when you completed the Personal Health Inventory. Pick one or two Whole Health goals that are key to achieving at least one of the important things you identified in step 1. Write down your goals here. Remember to make sure that your goals are SMART—specific, measurable, achievable, relevant, and time-bound. No matter how tempting it is to jump in with both feet, limit yourself to three or fewer goals. You want to set yourself up for success, not get overwhelmed on the second day.

List your goals here:

Goal #1: ____________________

Goal #2: ____________________

Goal #3: ____________________

Once you have set your goals, identify your first step for each goal based on your Personal Health Inventory self-ratings. Don't feel discouraged if you rated yourself a 1 for some (or even all) domains. Don't start by thinking about how to get to a 5 now. Instead, write down what you can do to move from a 1 to a 2 or a 2 to a 3. Recognizing the gaps between your current state and your desired future self is crucial for reducing low back pain. Keep in mind that this process is incremental. For example, suppose one of your goals is to walk a mile with your dog daily. You know that increased movement is essential to make that happen, so you add this to your goal list. You aim to walk five thousand steps daily, but you are currently spending much of your time sitting at work and at home. Start small. Use your smartphone or smartwatch to track your daily step count.

After several days of "baseline data," commit to walking a hundred steps farther each day. Or start with ten steps if a hundred is too much. Stay focused on moving in the right direction, even if your daily improvements are small. You will be surprised at how quickly your body adapts to your new activity level and gets stronger.

Once movement is a regular part of your life, you may see additional opportunities to address your low back pain. For instance, consider adding a ten-minute meditation to your daily routine. Numerous apps are available. Examples include Insight Timer, Calm, Headspace, and Peloton. On the first day, add daily meditation to your Action Plan and download the app you chose. On the second day, read the introductory information and sign up for a free trial. The next day, choose a short meditation exercise that is a good match with one of your Back Factors, such as help with sleeping or anxiety. Figure out what time of the day works best to schedule in ten uninterrupted minutes. Pick a location in your home or somewhere else you can sit comfortably. Commit to meditating for ten minutes a day every day for a week. Meditate for ten minutes a day for one week. Assess how things are going after you have met that goal. Is ten minutes too much or not enough time? Does the time of day and location you are using to meditate work for you? Begin experimenting with different meditation practices. There are literally thousands of options when it comes to guided meditation—don't give up before you find one that works for you.

Self-empowerment is believing in your ability to control your choices and take life-changing actions. You create space for that control by identifying what matters most to you and leveraging your strengths to overcome obstacles. While belief is the first thing, acting on those beliefs requires resilience and sustained motivation.

Here is how Jon, whom you met in chapter 5, and my friend Kate, whom you will meet shortly, developed their Action Plans. The first five basic steps were the same for both.

Step 1: Commit to change.

Step 2: Identify modifiable Back Factors.

Step 3: Link treatment approaches to Back Factors.

Step 4: Identify healthcare professionals who match treatment approaches.

Step 5: Complete the Action Plan template.

Remember that Jon's Back Factors were stress, ONTs, standing for long periods, and weak back muscles. Based on the patient flow diagram, he had several treatment options. He chose CBT and talk therapy to address his ONTs and anxiety. He chose exercise and mindfulness to address his anxiety and stress. And he chose spinal manipulation to address pain due to tight back muscles. Since a chiropractor provides spinal manipulation and exercise guidance, he decided to start with a chiropractor.

Here is a copy of Jon's Action Plan.

Whole Health Domains	Goals		
	Goal #1	**Goal #2**	**Goal #3**
	Build Core Strength and Stability	**Address Anxiety/ Stress/ONTs**	**Address Tight Back Muscles**
Moving the Body	• Work out at the gym 3x per week • Play pickleball regularly	• Go for a long walk with his dog at least once per day	• Walk 10K steps daily

Whole Health Domains	Goals		
	Goal #1	**Goal #2**	**Goal #3**
	Build Core Strength and Stability	**Address Anxiety/ Stress/ONTs**	**Address Tight Back Muscles**
Recharge		• Schedule regular alone time • Put down the smartphone at least an hour before bedtime	
Food and Drink		• Focus on healthy eating even when feeling stressed or experiencing a low back pain exacerbation	
Personal Development		• Read the book *10% Happier*, by Dan Harris • More clearly communicate career goals to the supervisor at work	• Download the Calm app and commit to meditating at least ten minutes each day • Actually meditate ten minutes each day

Whole Health Domains	Goals		
	Goal #1	**Goal #2**	**Goal #3**
	Build Core Strength and Stability	**Address Anxiety/ Stress/ONTs**	**Address Tight Back Muscles**
Family, Friends, and Coworkers	• Join a pickleball league with fiancé	• Share more about low back pain and mental health struggles with family and close friends	
Spirit and Soul		• Daily mindfulness meditation • Attend church regularly on Sunday mornings	
Surroundings		• Spend more time with family and friends	• Quit part-time job at the sporting goods store
Power of the Mind		• Complete Personal Health Inventory • Work on reframing ONTs	

Whole Health Domains	Goals		
	Goal #1	**Goal #2**	**Goal #3**
	Build Core Strength and Stability	**Address Anxiety/ Stress/ONTs**	**Address Tight Back Muscles**
Professional Care	• Schedule and keep five workout sessions with a personal trainer experienced in working with people living with low back pain	• Schedule and keep appointments with a psychologist trained in CBT 2x per month • Schedule and keep biweekly sessions with a health coach to discuss personal development	• Schedule and keep appointments with a chiropractor as needed to manage pain and increase physical functioning

As Jon developed his plan, he realized it was impossible to do everything at once. He fit the components of his Action Plan into his life sequentially, making adjustments to both his plan and his life as he went. The steps in the gray boxes are the ones he started with, adding the others over time.

Now, meet Kate.

Kate was one of the first people I met when I set out to learn to write like a real person rather than a scientist. We traveled two and a half hours together in the back of an Uber to attend a writing retreat held on an uninhabited island off the coast of Maine. When Kate started having low back pain a couple of years later, she expected to return to normal in a day or two. Instead, her pain was still there a few weeks later. She tried taking more and more Advil, sleeping on a heating pad, and buying new, more supportive shoes. When none of these strategies worked, she knew it was time to be more proactive, especially since she was also experiencing some depression. She called me and I introduced her to Whole Health.

Here is a copy of Kate's Action Plan.

Whole Health Domains	Goals		
	Goal #1	**Goal #2**	**Goal #3**
	Build Core Strength	**Address Depression**	**Increase Sense of Self-Empowerment**
Moving the Body	• Follow home PT regimen from Ann	• Go to an EarlyBirds Club event at Beat Kitchen	• Get up early and tackle one hard thing (exercise, chore) before breakfast
Recharge	• Restart a yoga practice	• Schedule a monthly massage	• Before watching TV, read at least one chapter or write a letter to a friend
Food and Drink		• Reduce alcohol use further	
Personal Development		• Have a gratitude journal for daily documentation	• Create a "Did It" Diary: Track daily accomplishments and recognize daily successes

Whole Health Domains	Goals		
	Goal #1	Goal #2	Goal #3
	Build Core Strength	Address Depression	Increase Sense of Self-Empowerment
Family, Friends, and Coworkers	• Join the rowing club with Nancy	• Engage friends in Chicago: Renata, Carol, Lisa, Nancy	• Send one letter a week to a friend, "Just Because"
Spirit and Soul	• Volunteer at Nourishing Hope (lifting and unloading boxes)	• Join an amateur choir at St. Luke's	
Surroundings	• During work, keep moving, lifting, and bending during the day	• Limit smartphone time to under three hours daily	• Create a safe, comfortable space in the office for work and play
Power of the Mind		• Set a timer for a bad mood or a sad feeling. Lean into the feeling and then let it go.	• Track feelings using the free How We Feel app
Professional Care	• Work with a trainer at the gym to safely build strength	• See licensed clinical social worker 1x per month to address depression	

Now it is time to develop your Action Plan.

There are many ways to approach this task. Here are some potential action steps using the same template as Jon and Kate.

1. List your goals at the top.
2. Review the nine Whole Health domains in chapter 6 if needed.
3. Add one or two Whole Health life changes that you commit to starting now.
4. Add one or more treatment approaches that you commit to using now.
5. List any healthcare professionals needed to help you reach your goals under Professional Care.

Whole Health Domains	Goals		
	Goal #1	Goal #2	Goal #3
Moving the Body			

Whole Health Domains	Goals		
	Goal #1	Goal #2	Goal #3
Recharge			
Food and Drink			
Personal Development			
Family, Friends, and Coworkers			

Whole Health Domains	Goals		
	Goal #1	Goal #2	Goal #3
Spirit and Soul			
Surroundings			
Power of the Mind			
Professional Care			

Step 5: Take Action

Once your Action Plan is complete, it is time for the hard part: taking action.

Getting Started

Jon got started by taping his Action Plan to his bathroom mirror, so it was the first and last thing he looked at every day. Seeing things in writing was affirming for him. He also added his action steps to his phone calendar to stay focused on his purpose. You already know from reading chapter 6 what a significant impact this had on Jon's low back pain and his life.

Kate shared her Action Plan with her friends and her physical therapist to get their feedback and support. At the time I am writing this book, she is on the third iteration of her ninety-day Action Plan. She is not as self-conscious at the gym. Her clothes fit differently. Her depressive thoughts are fainter than before. She still has low back pain sometimes. "However," she says, "I don't dwell on ONTs, go shopping online for wheelchairs, or spend days in bed with the curtains drawn. Instead, I lift weights in the gym, see my physical therapist when needed, and keep a gratitude journal. There is more change that I'd like to see in my life, but my Action Plan keeps me focused on the things that are important to me and the actions I need to take to make those things happen."

What Jon and Kate have both learned is that it doesn't matter how big or small their goals are. What matters is that those goals align with your overall life objectives, that they are achievable, and that you take action to achieve them.

Track Your Progress

An essential part of taking action is to track your progress over time. There are several reasons why. Tracking will help you determine if your Action Plan is working. You may need to add new treatment options or change direction entirely. Tracking your progress will also keep you motivated. Imagine that right before you initiated your Action Plan, you rated your low back pain as 9 on a 0–10 pain scale. After a few weeks of committing to, developing, and implementing your Action Plan, you have a day when you don't feel like doing your stretching exercises and going for a walk. Your pain is a little worse than it was the day before, and it doesn't seem like you are getting any better. You complete the pain scale again without looking at your old score, and rate your pain as a 5. When you compare the two scores, you realize that even if you have hit a plateau, your pain is significantly lower than it was when you started. You decide to exercise and go on that walk. Maybe in another three weeks, your pain level will be down to 3.

You can track your progress using the same three-question form I use to monitor patient progress in my research. It is called the PEG (pain, enjoyment of life, and general activity) scale. Using numbers from 0 to 10, answer the following three questions. For question 1, 0 means "no pain," and 10 means "pain as bad as you can imagine." For questions 2 and 3, 0 means "does not interfere," and 10 means "completely interferes."

1. What number best describes your pain on average in the past week?

   No pain **Pain as bad as you can imagine**

   ○0 ○1 ○2 ○3 ○4 ○5 ○6 ○7 ○8 ○9 ○10

2. What number best describes how, during the past week, pain has interfered with your enjoyment of life?

   Does not interfere **Completely interferes**

   ○0 ○1 ○2 ○3 ○4 ○5 ○6 ○7 ○8 ○9 ○10

3. What number best describes how, during the past week, pain has interfered with your general activity?

Does not interfere **Completely interferes**

o0 o1 o2 o3 o4 o5 o6 o7 o8 o9 o10

If all three of these questions apply to the pain management goals you have set for yourself, use all three. If only one or two apply, focus on those.

It is also important to track any side effects experienced from the treatments you are using. Examples range from temporary soreness after spinal manipulation to dizziness from taking prescription medication. List each side effect and then rate how bothersome that symptom has been in the past week, using a 0–5 scale, with 0 being not at all bothersome and 5 being extremely bothersome.

List your side effects here:

Side Effect #1 ______________________________

o0 o1 o2 o3 o4 o5

Side Effect #2 ______________________________

o0 o1 o2 o3 o4 o5

Side Effect #3 ______________________________

o0 o1 o2 o3 o4 o5

Side Effect #4 ______________________________

o0 o1 o2 o3 o4 o5

As you have already learned, the risk of side effects exists with every available treatment approach for low back pain. Often, side effects go away on their own in just a few days or weeks. Others can worsen or become more bothersome over time. Tracking side effect information and comparing it to your low back pain symptoms provides valuable insights for both you and your healthcare professional. Here is an example of how this works. Suppose your pain level decreases from an 8 to a 3, and you rate the dizziness from the medication that helped make that happen at a 2. Using that medication might be right for you. However, if your pain level stays the same or only decreases to a 7, and your dizziness is rated at a 5, you might need to try a different treatment approach.

Don't forget about your Whole Health Personal Health Inventory. Filling it out every three months can help you track progress and determine next steps.

Step 6: Take Action

Your Action Plan is not set in stone. Many people with low back pain find relief within a week or two after initiating their first treatment choice. Others may need to try an alternative approach or combine multiple treatments. Still others learn to manage their pain—while it is still present to some extent, the pain does not define who they are or how they live their lives. If whatever tracking system you use shows you are improving, keep doing what you are doing. If not, switch to another recommended treatment. For example, try spinal manipulation instead of massage. You can also combine treatments to address multiple Back Factors—maybe add mindfulness to spinal manipulation and exercise. Combinations of treatments can be especially helpful if you have had pain for longer than a few weeks. Here is Kate's final observation: "Creating and executing on my Action Plan was not a 'set it and forget it' process. I have had to tweak the plan over time. Just looking back over the past year, I see that I want to try new things (and maybe harder things) now that I've met some of my goals. The initial plan was exactly what I needed at the time, and now I want to do more."

Creating a personalized care plan is about more than just managing pain—it's about taking control of your health and empowering yourself to make informed decisions. By understanding the underlying Back Factors contributing to your pain, exploring a range of treatment options, and working with healthcare professionals who are the right fit for you, you can build an Action Plan that supports both immediate relief and long-term well-being.

Remember, there is no one-size-fits-all solution. It takes patience, persistence, and the right tools to navigate your low back pain journey confidently. Stay committed, stay informed, and trust yourself—you are the best advocate in your journey to healing.

On a final note, as the Whole Health approach emphasizes, it is vital to surround yourself with people who can support your goals. These people may be family and friends but may also include healthcare clinicians or other professionals you consult for help with your low back pain, like yoga instructors or massage therapists.

Key Takeaways

- ✓ Choose your treatment approaches based on your specific Back Factors.
- ✓ Determine if you need help from a health professional, what kind of help you need, and who the right person is to provide that help.
- ✓ Develop your Action Plan by outlining the steps needed to make forward progress. You can do this on your own or with the help of a health professional.
- ✓ Implement your plan by setting specific goals and tracking your progress.
- ✓ Make changes when needed.

chapter 23

Final Key Takeaways

You have reached the end of *Take Your Back Back*. You have come far—not just in reading these pages but in your willingness to seek new answers, challenge old beliefs, and take charge of your healing journey. Low back pain is one of the most common and frustrating health challenges worldwide. It doesn't have to be that way. You now have the knowledge you need to embark on a path toward less pain, better physical functioning, and more optimal health. You also have a road map to help you translate this knowledge into practical action steps. Here are a few key takeaways to keep in mind along the way.

1. *You Are Not Alone.*

Your experience with low back pain is unique. However, the research, patients, and healthcare professionals you were introduced to within these pages clearly demonstrate that you are not alone. Many people—others experiencing low back pain, family members, friends, colleagues, and a wide range of healthcare professionals—can offer support regardless of where you are on your low back pain journey.

2. *Whole Health Matters.*

Tackling low back pain is more about "what matters to you" than "what is the matter with you." Healing is about more than just your back. The Whole Health model encourages you to look at your life from a broad perspective—your movement, nutrition, sleep, relationships, personal development, and the power of the mind. By confronting common myths, identifying your "Back Factors," and setting SMART goals, you can create an Action Plan that is specific to who you are and what you want from this stage in your life, and that addresses the physical, emotional, social, environmental, and spiritual aspects of low back pain.

3. Consistent Self-Management Is Key.

You are the expert on your own low back pain. Self-management, manifested through resilience, self-empowerment, and sustained motivation, puts you in charge of your low back pain journey. Whether it's starting a walking routine, practicing mindfulness, or turning to a healthcare professional for help, small, consistent actions add up to meaningful change. Remember, healing your low back pain boils down to making decisions and then taking the next right action step. Decisions that are difficult at first and work that seems complicated ultimately become routine. Making decisions, pushing through the initial awkwardness of trying new things, and recommitting over and over again to stick with new habits requires focused effort.

Take my low back pain story as an example. I finally found the help I needed after a year of struggling through the pain. While my chiropractor and my psychologist played essential roles in that process, I needed to make significant changes in my life to support my healing journey. I had to become more physically active, discover meditation, and confront my fears. These changes were challenging at first. However, thirty-five years later, they are woven into the fabric of my life. I still have mild to moderate low back pain on occasion. The pain serves as a reminder to get back into my walking routine, assess my stress levels, practice meditation, remember to breathe, and schedule a visit with a chiropractor, an acupuncturist, or a massage therapist. The pain never gets too bad or lasts very long because I now have the knowledge and skills to manage my low back pain rather than it managing me.

4. There Is No One-Size-Fits-All Solution.

What works for Jon or Kate's low back pain may not work for you. You may need to consider multiple treatment approaches, either sequentially or in combination. Your journey will have ups and downs. Expect setbacks. They are a regular part of the low back pain journey. Remember to keep moving forward and adapt your Action Plan as needed. Keep in mind that what works best for you right now may not be what your mind and body need six months or a year from now. As your goals change, adjust your plan. These adjustments are an important part of the process.

5. Knowledge Is Power.

To help you on this journey, I have included recommendations for books throughout *Take Your Back Back* that can provide a deeper dive into specific topic areas. I have also suggested websites that link to informative videos, search engines for finding healthcare professionals in your area, and apps that can help you on your low back pain journey. You will find a list of these resources at the end of the book.

As you engage in the next phase of your low back pain journey, keep in mind that new knowledge is constantly evolving. Treatments that are considered experimental today may be shown to be safe and effective in the future. The opposite may also be true. The resources found in this book will evolve as well. Some might already be out of date by the time you read these words. In addition, there is always more to learn. Future discoveries will lead to better ways of diagnosing low back pain, new treatment approaches, and changes in health plan payment policies.

Here are a few ways to stay current:

- Set Google Alerts for topics or authors you want to track.
- Visit the National Center for Complementary and Integrative Health at the National Institutes of Health website and sign up for their mailing list.
- Visit my website for the latest low back pain research and insights into what this new knowledge might mean for you.

As you close this book, remember that healing your low back pain is a journey that only you can lead. Your low back pain does not define you. Rather, it is your persistence, your choices, and your actions that define you.

It is time to take your back back:
one decision, one action, one day at a time.

Acknowledgments

I am so incredibly grateful to have not one, but two, of the best literary agents in the world. To Sheree Bykofsky, for believing in me before I believed in myself, and to Rita Rosenkranz, for pushing me to be a better writer and author. I am equally thankful to Lauren Marino, executive editor at Simon & Schuster. I knew during our very first call that Lauren was the right editor for *Take Your Back Back*. That feeling was only reinforced when I met editorial assistant Katie McClimon. All four of these women have been amazing to work with, and their guidance was essential to my writing process. Thanks also to copy editor Eileen G. Chetti, and to all the behind-the-scenes people at Simon & Schuster who helped make this book a reality.

Next, I would like to thank the many patients, healthcare professionals, and others who agreed to be interviewed for this book. In addition to those named in its pages, special thanks to Drs. Ben Kligler, Roger Chou, Nandan Lad, and Mark McClelland; acupuncturists Janet Schafer and Heather Bree; massage therapist Janet Kahn, and AHIP leaders Kate Berry and Chris Regal.

I would also like to thank the people who read this book in its entirety before it was submitted for publication and provided their expert advice, including Drs. Louis Sportelli, Robert Trager (double thanks to Dr. Trager for also helping with fact-checking), Robin Boineau, and Marion Couch.

My transition from scientific journal author to book author required a steep, iterative learning curve. For help along that journey, I am grateful to Darcey Witman and Wide Open Writing for teaching me what a writing prompt is and how to use one. I will never forget my WOW writing retreat, including the people I met there and the time I spent sitting alone at the top of a working lighthouse on an island off the coast of Maine, searching for my "voice." I am equally grateful to the organizers and my fellow participants at the Yale Writers Workshop (class of 2024), especially my workshop group. While there, I was introduced to the basics of the business part of writing, learned that "workshop" can be a verb, and how to hone my writing skills. I sent my first agent query letter from the Yale University library.

Early in this book's evolution, I imagined asking different people to write chapters while I served in an organizational and editorial capacity. In discussing this idea with friend and colleague Dr. Stacie Salsbury, she told me. "Christine, you have the expertise and the talent to write this book yourself. Even more importantly, you have a unique voice that the world needs to hear." Those words completely changed my perception of how this book might look and what I might be capable of doing. Thank you, Stacie.

A good book needs good editors before it can ever reach an agent or a publisher. Thanks to writing coach Maggie McReynolds, who taught me the basic template for writing prescriptive nonfiction and edited the earliest drafts of my first attempts at writing book chapters. Much later in the process, I am forever grateful to Scott DeGeest for doing his best to stamp out my passive voice and rein in my predilection for run-on sentences. This task sometimes required 100 or more comments per chapter.

Thanks to Geronimo Bejarano, PhD, now a postdoctoral fellow at the Harvard T.H. Chan School of Public Health, for being the best research assistant a person focused on low back pain could ever want.

You will meet my stepson, Jonathan Beck DeGeest, in this book. A special thanks goes out to him for sharing his low back pain story and Whole Health journey with me, and with all of you.

I am also grateful to Kate Faber. Kate is a member of the First Four Writing Group, along with fellow writers Tiffany Dugan and Gabrielle McGhee. The four of us connected during the WOW retreat in Maine and subsequently spent two hours writing together virtually every week for more than two years. Kate shared her Whole Health Journey with you in this book and also helped me with editing and keeping me organized on the administrative aspects of writing a book. Special thanks also to writing friends Siohban

Armstrong and Dr. Diane Solomon. I might have been able to write this book without the support and encouragement of these five women, but it would not have been nearly as much fun.

Thanks go to the amazing people who provided their expertise in yoga and exercise instruction as I wrote the first three chapters of part 2 of *Take Your Back Back*. Nathan Goertz, Christy Buffington, Tanya Witman, and Mauricio Nunez helped choose the yoga poses (Tanya) and exercises (Nathan, Christy, and Mauricio) described in the book, led me step by step through each pose and exercise, and served as the models for all the photographs. I am also grateful to Reed Peterson for taking the photographs, to Showalter Johnson for making them perfect, and to MUSCO Lighting, Jeanie Beiri, and Joe Crookham for donating the studio space to take the photographs.

Special thanks go to Dan Humphreys for creating the illustrations in this book. I had no idea (and I am sure Dan did not either) what an iterative process this would be as we worked with Simon & Schuster to get everything exactly right. I am also grateful to my brother Jeff Horon. Jeff created the illustration I used to explain the Take Your Back Back Action Plan to my agents and editors. I also extend my thanks to Elissa Allen for doing an amazing job formatting my original book proposal and my manuscript before submission, as well as for her editorial help all along the way.

I am grateful to the dedicated clinicians and administrators at Duke University School of Medicine, whose stories about caring for patients with low back pain inspired me to write this book. You will meet many of them in these pages. Special thanks also to my fellow research "MSKTeers," Drs. Steve George, Adam Goode, Trevor Lentz, and Lindsay Ballengee, as well as the Spine Health Executive (SHE) team, Sara Holleran, Jennie Wahl, Kayla Daniels, and Damien Lett.

Despite the many people involved in writing a book, it is still a scary, somewhat lonely journey, especially for a first-time author. I am grateful every day for the encouragement I received from my family—Randy, David, Dan, Nathan, Hanna, Jon, Sarah, Ian, and Lynn—and their patience as I committed almost every waking moment for almost three years to researching low back pain, writing about low back pain, or talking about low back pain. The same goes to members of "The Wood Hood"—Joe, Jeanie, Neal, Marcia, Jennifer, and Nate. Finally, thanks to my mother, Elizabeth Wisner Horon, who passed on to me both her love of reading and talent for writing.

Resources

Chapter 5:

Introduction to Whole Health

Website:

Veterans Health Administration Whole Health Resources: https://www.va.gov/wholehealth/

Book:

Talking Back: How to Overcome Chronic Back Pain and Rebuild Your Life by Dr. Rowland Hazard

Chapter 6:

Whole Health and Low Back Pain

Personal Development

Book:

10% Happier: How I Tamed the Voice in My Head, Reduced Stress Without Losing My Edge, and Found Self-Health That Actually Works by Dan Harris

Food and Drink

Books:

The Science-Backed Anti-Inflammatory Diet for Beginners by Drs. Yasmine Elamir and William Grist

Super Gut: A Four-Week Plan to Reprogram Your Microbiome, Restore Health, and Lose Weight by Dr. William Davis

Family, Friends, Coworkers, and Community

Book:

The Blue Zones by Dan Buettner

Chapter 7:

Self-Management

Resilience

Books:

The Artist's Way, by Julia Cameron

The Book of Alchemy, by Suleika Jaouad

Website:

Mayo Clinic free thirty-day gratitude program: https://www.mayoclinichealthsystem.org/wellness/gratitude

Sustained Motivation

Books:

Atomic Habits by James Clear

Scarcity Brain: Fix Your Craving Mindset and Rewire Your Habits to Thrive with Enough by Michael Easter

The Power of Discipline: How to Use Self Control and Mental Toughness to Achieve Your Goals by Daniel Walter

Tiny Habits: The Small Changes That Change Everything by B. J. Fogg, PhD

Do the Hard Things First by Scott Allan

Chapter 8:

An Introduction to Exercise

App:

Peloton

Chapter 9:

Yoga Poses

Books:

The Yoga Bible: The Definitive Guide to Yoga Postures by Christina Brown

Perfectly Imperfect: The Art and Soul of Yoga Practice by Baron Baptiste

Chapter 11:

Common Self-Care Treatments

Website:

How to Use a TENS Unit: https://uihc.org/health-topics/transcutaneous-electrical-nerve-stimulator-tens)

Chapter 12:

Body-Based Treatment Approaches

Book:

The Web That Has No Weaver by Ted J. Kaptchuk

Chapter 13:

Mind-Based Approaches—Mindfulness Meditation

Books:

Meditations for Mortals: Four Weeks to Embrace Your Limitations and Make Time for What Counts by Oliver Burkeman

Think Like a Monk: Train Your Mind for Peace and Purpose by Jay Shetty

Apps:

Calm

Headspace

Insight Timer

Websites:

Duke Health and Well-Being Program: https://dhwprograms.dukehealth.org/programs-training/public/experiencing-mindfulness/

Harvard University Mindfulness and Meditation: https://wellness.huhs.harvard.edu/your-wellbeing/mindfulness-and-meditation/

Stanford Healthcare Mindfulness-Based Stress Reduction (MBSR): https://stanfordhealthcare.org/events/mindfulness-based-stress-reduction-mbsr.html

Chapter 14:

Mind-Based Approaches—Psychological Treatments

Books:

Mindfulness for Beginners by Dr. Jon Kabat-Zinn

Full Catastrophe Living by Dr. Jon Kabat-Zinn

The Pain Management Workbook by Rachel Zoffness

Websites:

Rachel Zoffness Pain Management Resources: https://www.zoffness.com/resources

Empowered Relief Provider Directory: https://empoweredrelief.stanford.edu

Free self-guided CBT pain program: https://www.PainTrainer.org

Chapter 15:

Prescription Medications

Websites:

Opioid Use Disorder or Addiction: https://www.hhs.gov/opioids/index.html

Opioid Use Treatment: https://findtreatment.gov

Call Line:

Opioid Use Treatment: 1-800-662-HELP (4357)

Important note regarding sources for chapters 18–20

Following are several searchable directories to locate specific healthcare professionals in your area. Keep in mind that these websites are managed by professional organizations that list their members or others who may pay a fee to be included. You cannot assume that the listed healthcare professionals have been vetted for quality of care or that their credentials have been confirmed.

Chapter 18:

Finding the Right Healthcare Professional

Websites:

American Chiropractic Association: https://handsdownbetter.org/find-a-doctor/

WebMD: https://doctor.webmd.com/providers/specialty/chiropractor

American Academy of Orthopaedic Manual Physical Therapists: https://aaompt.org/Main/Main/Member_Resources/Find-A-Fellow.aspx

American Board of Physical Therapy Specialists web portal: https://specialization.apta.org/find-a-specialist **(Note: Select Orthopaedic and hit search)**

American Physical Therapy Association: https://www.choosept.com/find-a-pt

American Psychological Association: https://locator.apa.org/

Finding a Psychologist: https://www.psychologytoday.com/us

Chapter 19:

Medical Professionals

Websites:

American Board of Medical Specialties Website (for Patients): https://www.certificationmatters.org

American Osteopathic Association: https://findado.osteopathic.org/

Chapter 20:

Other Professionals Who Can Help with Your Low Back Pain

Websites:

Yoga Alliance Directory: https://yogaalliance.org/find-a-yoga-teacher/

National Board Certified Health & Wellness Coaches Directory: https://members.nbhwc.org/search/

National Massage Therapy Association Directory: https://www.amtamassage.org/find-massage-therapist/

National Certification Commission for Acupuncture and Oriental Medicine Directory: https://www.nccaom.org/find-a-practitioner-directory/

Chapter 21:

Advocate for Yourself

Websites:

ProPublica Claims File Process: https://projects.propublica.org/claimfile/

US Pain Foundation: https://uspainfoundation.org/

Chapter 22:

The Take Your Back Back Action Plan

Food

Apps:

Noom

EatRightNow

MyFitnessPal

Mental Health

App:

How We Feel

Staying Current

Websites:

National Center for Complementary and Integrative Health: https://www.nccih.nih.gov

Dr. Christine Goertz: https://cgoertzllc.com

References

Introduction

Becker A, Held H, Redaelli M, et al. "Low Back Pain in Primary Care: Costs of Care and Prediction of Future Health Care Utilization." *Spine* 35 (18) (2010): 1714–20. doi:10.1097/brs.0b013e3181cd656f.

"The Lancet Series Call to Action to Reduce Low Value Care for Low Back Pain: An Update." *Pain* 161, Suppl 1 (1) (2020): S57–S64. doi:10.1097/j.pain.0000000000001869.

Chou R, Baisden J, Carragee EJ, Resnick DK, Shaffer WO, and Loeser JD. "Surgery for Low Back Pain: A Review of the Evidence for an American Pain Society Clinical Practice Guideline." *Spine* 34 (10) (2009): 1094–1109. doi:10.1097/BRS.0b013e3181a105fc.

Chou R, Loeser JD, Owens DK, et al. "Interventional Therapies, Surgery, and Interdisciplinary Rehabilitation for Low Back Pain: An Evidence-Based Clinical Practice Guideline from the American Pain Society." *Spine* 34 (10) (2009):1066–77. doi:10.1097/BRS.0b013e3181a139 0d.

Chou R, Qaseem A, Owens DK, and Shekelle P. "Clinical Guidelines Committee of the American College of Physicians. Diagnostic Imaging for Low Back Pain: Advice for High-Value Health Care from the American College of Physicians." *Annals of Internal Medicine* 154 (3) (2011): 181–89. doi:10.7326/0003-4819-154-3-201102010-00008.

Curatolo M, Rundell SD, Gold LS, et al. "Long-Term Effectiveness of Epidural Steroid Injections After New Episodes of Low Back Pain in Older Adults." *European Journal of Pain*. Published online May 23, 2022. doi:10.1002/ejp.1975.

Darlow B, Dean S, Perry M, Mathieson F, Baxter GD, and Dowell A. "Easy to Harm, Hard to Heal: Patient Views About the Back. *Spine* 40 (11) (2015): 842–50. doi:10.1097/BRS.0000000000000901.

Darlow B, Dowell A, Baxter GD, Mathieson F, Perry M, and Dean S. "The Enduring Impact of What Clinicians Say to People with Low Back Pain." *Annals of Family Medicine* 11 (6) (2013): 527–34. doi:10.1370/afm.1518.

Dieleman JL, Cao J, Chapin A, et al. "US Health Care Spending by Payer and Health Condition, 1996–2016." *JAMA* 323 (9) (2020): 863–84. doi:10.1001/jama.2020.0734.

Ding Y and Liu C. "Alternative Payment Models and Physician Treatment Decisions: Evidence from Lower Back Pain." *Journal of Health Economics* 80 (2021): 102548. doi:10.1016/j.jhealeco.2021.102548.

Finley CR, Chan DS, Garrison S, et al. "What Are the Most Common Conditions in Primary Care?" *Canadian Family Physician* 64 (11) (2018): 832–40.

GBD 2016. "Disease and Injury Incidence and Prevalence Collaborators. Global, Regional, and National Incidence, Prevalence, and Years Lived with Disability for 328 Diseases and Injuries for 195 Countries, 1990–2016: A Systematic Analysis for the Global Burden of Disease Study 2016." *Lancet* 390 (10100) (2017): 1211–59. doi:10.1016/S0140-6736 (17)32154-2.

Hall AM, Aubrey-Bassler K, Thorne B, and Maher CG. "Do Not Routinely Offer Imaging for Uncomplicated Low Back Pain." *BMJ* 372:n291 (2021). doi:10.1136/bmj.n291.

Hartvigsen J, Hancock MJ, Kongsted A, et al. "What Low Back Pain Is and Why We Need to Pay Attention." *Lancet* 391 (10137) (2018): 2356–67. doi:10.1016/S0140-6736(18)30480-X.

Hong AS, Ross-Degnan D, Zhang F, and Wharam JF. "Small Decline in Low-Value Back Imaging Associated with the 'Choosing Wisely' Campaign, 2012–14." *Health Affairs Project Hope* 36 (4) (2017): 671–79. doi:10.1377/hlthaff.2016.1263.

Hoy D, Bain C, Williams G, et al. "A Systematic Review of the Global Prevalence of Low Back Pain." *Arthritis & Rheumatology* 64 (6) (2012): 2028–37. doi:10.1002/art.34347.

Jones CMP, Day RO, Koes BW, et al. "Opioid Analgesia for Acute Low Back Pain and Neck Pain (the OPAL Trial): A Randomised Placebo-Controlled Trial." *Lancet* 402 (10398) (2023): 304–12. doi:10.1016/S0140-6736 (23)00404-X.

Qaseem A, Wilt TJ, McLean RM, Forciea MA. and Clinical Guidelines Committee of the American College of Physicians. "Noninvasive Treatments for Acute, Subacute, and Chronic Low Back Pain: A Clinical Practice Guideline from the American College of Physicians." *Annals of Internal Medicine* 166 (7) (2017): 514–30. doi:10.7326/M16-2367.

Rainville J, Smeets RJEM, Bendix T, Tveito TH, Poiraudeau S, and Indahl AJ. "Fear-Avoidance Beliefs and Pain Avoidance in Low Back Pain—Translating Research into Clinical Practice." *Spine Journal* 11 (9) (2011): 895–903. doi:10.1016/j.spinee.2011.08.006.

Saragiotto BT, Machado GC, Ferreira ML, Pinheiro MB, Abdel Shaheed C, and Maher CG. "Paracetamol for Low Back Pain." *Cochrane Database of Systematic Reviews* (6) (2016): CD012230. doi:10.1002/14651858.CD012230.

Staal JB, de Bie R, de Vet HC, Hildebrandt J, and Nelemans P. "Injection Therapy for Subacute and Chronic Low Back Pain." *Cochrane Database of Systematic Reviews* (3) (2008): CD001824. doi:10.1002/14651858.CD001824.pub3.

St. Sauver JL, Warner DO, Yawn BP, et al. "Why Do Patients Visit their Doctors? Assessing the Most Prevalent Conditions in a Defined US Population." *Mayo Clinic Proceedings* 88 (1) (2013): 56–67. doi:10.1016/j.mayocp.2012.08.020.

"WHO Guideline for Non-Surgical Management of Chronic Primary Low Back Pain in Adults in Primary and Community Care Settings." World Health Organization. Accessed December 15, 2023. https://www.who.int/publications-detail-redirect/9789240081789.

Wu A, March L, Zheng X, et al. "Global Low Back Pain Prevalence and Years Lived with Disability from 1990 to 2017: Estimates from the Global Burden of Disease Study 2017." *Annals of Translational Medicine* 8 (6) (2020). doi:10.21037/atm.2020.02.175.

Yavin D, Casha S, Wiebe S, et al. "Lumbar Fusion for Degenerative Disease: A Systematic Review and Meta-Analysis." *Neurosurgery* 80 (5) (2017):701–15. doi:10.1093/neuros/nyw162.

Zadro J, O'Keeffe M, and Maher C. "Do Physical Therapists Follow Evidence-Based Guidelines When Managing Musculoskeletal Conditions? Systematic Review." *BMJ Open* 9 (10) (2019): e032329. doi:10.1136/bmjopen-2019-032329.

Chapter 1

Qaseem A, Wilt TJ, McLean RM, Forciea MA, and Clinical Guidelines Committee of the American College of Physicians. "Noninvasive Treatments for Acute, Subacute, and Chronic Low Back

Pain: A Clinical Practice Guideline from the American College of Physicians." *Annals of Internal Medicine* 166 (7) (2017): 514–30. doi:10.7326/M16-2367.

Stevans JM, Delitto A, Khoja SS, et al. "Risk Factors Associated with Transition from Acute to Chronic Low Back Pain in US Patients Seeking Primary Care." *JAMA Network Open* 4 (2) (2021): e2037371. doi:10.1001/jamanetworkopen.2020.37371.

"WHO Guideline for Non-Surgical Management of Chronic Primary Low Back Pain in Adults in Primary and Community Care Settings." World Health Organization. Accessed December 15, 2023. https://www.who.int/publications-detail-redirect/9789240081789.

Chapter 2

Artus M, van der Windt DA, Jordan KP, and Hay EM. "Low Back Pain Symptoms Show a Similar Pattern of Improvement Following a Wide Range of Primary Care Treatments: A Systematic Review of Randomized Clinical Trials." *Rheumatology* 49 (12) (2010): 2346–56. doi:10.1093/rheumatology/keq245.

Buchbinder R, van Tulder M, Öberg B, et al. "Low Back Pain: A Call for Action." *Lancet* 391 (10137) (2018): 2384–88. doi:10.1016/S0140-6736 (18)30488-4.

Cashin AG, Wand BM, O'Connell NE, et al. "Pharmacological Treatments for Low Back Pain in Adults: An Overview of Cochrane Reviews. *Cochrane Database of Systematic Reviews* (4) (2023). doi:10.1002/14651858.CD013815.pub2.

Choo EK, Charlesworth CJ, Gu Y, Livingston CJ, and McConnell KJ. "Increased Use of Complementary and Alternative Therapies for Back Pain Following Statewide Medicaid Coverage Changes in Oregon." *Journal of General Internal Medicine* 36 (3) (2021): 676–82. doi:10.1007/s11606-020-06352-6.

Curatolo M, Rundell SD, Gold LS, et al. "Long-Term Effectiveness of Epidural Steroid Injections After New Episodes of Low Back Pain in Older Adults." *European Journal of Pain*. Published online May 23, 2022. doi:10.1002/ejp.1975.

Delitto A, Patterson CG, Stevans JM, et al. "Stratified Care to Prevent Chronic Low Back Pain in High-Risk Patients: The TARGET Trial. A Multi-Site Pragmatic Cluster Randomized Trial. *eClinicalMedicine* 34 (2021). doi:10.1016/j.eclinm.2021.100795.

Ferreira GE, McLachlan AJ, Lin CWC, et al. "Efficacy and Safety of Antidepressants for the Treatment of Back Pain and Osteoarthritis: Systematic Review and Meta-Analysis." *BMJ* 372 (2021): m4825. doi:10.1136/bmj.m4825.

Jones CMP, Day RO, Koes BW, et al. "Opioid Analgesia for Acute Low Back Pain and Neck Pain (the OPAL Trial): A Randomised Placebo-Controlled Trial." *Lancet* 402 (10398) (2023): 304–12. doi:10.1016/S0140-6736 (23)00404-X.

Hartvigsen J, Kamper SJ, and French SD. "Low-Value Care in Musculoskeletal Health Care: Is There a Way Forward?" *Pain Practice* 22 (Suppl 2) (2022): 65–70. doi:10.1111/papr.13142.

Hayden JA, Ogilvie R, Kashif S, et al. "Exercise Treatments for Chronic Low Back Pain: A Network Meta-Analysis." *Cochrane Database of Systematic Reviews* (6) (2023). doi:10.1002/14651858.CD015608.

Heyward J, Jones CM, Compton WM, et al. "Coverage of Nonpharmacologic Treatments for Low Back Pain Among US Public and Private Insurers." *JAMA Network Open* 1 (6) (2018): e183044. doi:10.1001/jamanetworkopen.2018.3044.

Krebs EE, Gravely A, Nugent S, et al. "Effect of Opioid vs. Nonopioid Medications on Pain-Related Function in Patients with Chronic Back Pain or Hip or Knee Osteoarthritis Pain: The SPACE Randomized Clinical Trial." *JAMA* 319 (9) (2018): 872–82. doi:10.1001/jama.2018.0899.

Lentz TA, Rhon DI, and George SZ. "Predicting Opioid Use, Increased Health Care Utilization and High Costs for Musculoskeletal Pain: What Factors Mediate Pain Intensity and Disability?" *Journal of Pain* 21 (1–2) (2020): 135–45. doi:10.1016/j.jpain.2019.06.004.

Qaseem A, Wilt TJ, McLean RM, Forciea MA, and Clinical Guidelines Committee of the American College of Physicians. "Noninvasive Treatments for Acute, Subacute, and Chronic Low Back Pain: A Clinical Practice Guideline from the American College of Physicians." *Annals of Internal Medicine* 166 (7) (2017): 514–30. doi:10.7326/M16-2367.

Rubinstein SM, Zoete A de, Middelkoop M van, Assendelft WJJ, Boer MR de, and Tulder MW van. "Benefits and Harms of Spinal Manipulative Therapy for the Treatment of Chronic Low Back Pain: Systematic Review and Meta-Analysis of Randomised Controlled Trials." *BMJ* 364 (2019): l689. doi:10.1136/bmj.l689.

Schreijenberg M, Koes BW, and Lin CWC. "Guideline Recommendations on the Pharmacological Management of Non-Specific Low Back Pain in Primary Care—Is There a Need to Change?" *Expert Review of Clinical Pharmacology* 12 (2) (2019): 145–57. doi:10.1080/17512433.2019.1565992.

Stevans JM, Delitto A, Khoja SS, et al. "Risk Factors Associated with Transition from Acute to Chronic Low Back Pain in US Patients Seeking Primary Care." *JAMA Network Open* 4 (2) (2021): e2037371. doi:10.1001/jamanetworkopen.2020.37371.

Viana da Silva P, Kamper SJ, Robson E, et al. "'Myths and Facts' Education Is Comparable to 'Facts Only' for Recall of Back Pain Information but May Improve Fear-Avoidance Beliefs: An Embedded Randomized Trial." *Journal of Orthopaedic & Sports Physical Therapy*. Published online July 8, 2022: 1–29. doi:10.2519/jospt.2022.10989.

"WHO Guideline for Non-Surgical Management of Chronic Primary Low Back Pain in Adults in Primary and Community Care Settings." World Health Organization. Accessed December 15, 2023. https://www.who.int/publications-detail-redirect/9789240081789.

Chapter 3

Alhowimel A, AlOtaibi M, Radford K, and Coulson N. "Psychosocial Factors Associated with Change in Pain and Disability Outcomes in Chronic Low Back Pain Patients Treated by Physiotherapist: A Systematic Review. *SAGE Open Medicine* 6 (2018): 2050312118757387. doi:10.1177/2050312118757387.

Alzahrani H, Mackey M, Stamatakis E, Zadro JR, and Shirley D. "The Association Between Physical Activity and Low Back Pain: A Systematic Review and Meta-Analysis of Observational Studies." *Scientific Reports* 9 (1) (2019): 8244. doi:10.1038/s41598-019-44664-8.

Bourke MJ, Ferguson D, and Cooke M. "Patient Experiences of Self-Management for Chronic Low Back Pain: A Qualitative Study." *Physical Therapy & Rehabilitation Journal*. Published online March 30, 2022: pzac030. doi:10.1093/ptj/pzac030.

Briggs AM, Jordan JE, Buchbinder R, et al. "Health Literacy and Beliefs Among a Community Cohort with and Without Chronic Low Back Pain." *Pain* 150 (2) (2010): 275–83. doi:10.1016/j.pain.2010.04.031.

Campbell LC, Clauw DJ, and Keefe FJ. "Persistent Pain and Depression: A Biopsychosocial Perspective. *Biological Psychiatry* 54 (3) (2003): 399–409. doi:10.1016/s0006-3223 (03)00545-6.

Chou R, Qaseem A, Owens DK, Shekelle P, and Clinical Guidelines Committee of the American College of Physicians. "Diagnostic Imaging for Low Back Pain: Advice for High-Value Health Care from the American College of Physicians." *Annals of Internal Medicine* 154 (3) (2011): 181–89. doi:10.7326/0003-4819-154-3-201102010-00008.

Daoust R, Paquet J, Cournoyer A, et al. "Relationship Between Acute Pain Trajectories After an Emergency Department Visit and Chronic Pain: A Canadian Prospective Cohort Study." *BMJ Open*10 (12) (2020): e040390. doi:10.1136/bmjopen-2020-040390.

Delitto A, Patterson CG, Stevans JM, et al. "Stratified Care to Prevent Chronic Low Back Pain in High-Risk Patients: The TARGET Trial. A Multi-Site Pragmatic Cluster Randomized Trial." *eClinicalMedicine* 34 (2021). doi:10.1016/j.eclinm.2021.100795.

Engel GL. "The Need for a New Medical Model: A Challenge for Biomedicine." *Science* 196 (4286) (1977): 129–36. doi:10.1126/science.847460.

Ferreira PH, Ferreira ML, Maher CG, Refshauge KM, Latimer J, and Adams RD. "The Therapeutic Alliance Between Clinicians and Patients Predicts Outcome in Chronic Low Back Pain." *Physical Therapy & Rehabilitation Journal* 93 (4) (2013): 470–78. doi:10.2522/ptj.20120137.

Finucane LM, Downie A, Mercer C, et al. "International Framework for Red Flags for Potential Serious Spinal Pathologies." *Journal of Orthopaedic & Sports Physical Therapy* 50 (7) (2020): 350–72. doi:10.2519/jospt.2020.9971.

Gardner T, Refshauge K, McAuley J, Hübscher M, Goodall S, and Smith L. "Goal Setting Practice in Chronic Low Back Pain. What Is Current Practice and Is It Affected by Beliefs and Attitudes?" *Physiotherapy Theory and Practice* 34 (10) (2018): 795–805. doi:10.1080/09593985.2018.1425785.

Hartvigsen J, Hancock MJ, Kongsted A, et al. "What Low Back Pain Is and Why We Need to Pay Attention." *Lancet* 391 (10137) (2018): 2356–67. doi:10.1016/S0140-6736(18)30480-X.

Kamper SJ, Apeldoorn AT, Chiarotto A, et al. "Multidisciplinary Biopsychosocial Rehabilitation for Chronic Low Back Pain: Cochrane Systematic Review and Meta-Analysis." *BMJ* 350 (2015): h444. doi:10.1136/bmj.h444.

Karran EL, Grant AR, and Moseley GL. "Low Back Pain and the Social Determinants Of Health: A Systematic Review and Narrative Synthesis." *Pain* 161 (11) (2020): 2476–93. doi:10.1097/j.pain.0000000000001944.

Kreiner DS, Matz P, Bono CM, et al. "Guideline Summary Review: An Evidence-Based Clinical Guideline for the Diagnosis and Treatment of Low Back Pain." *Spine Journal* 20 (7) (2020): 998–1024. doi:10.1016/j.spinee.2020.04.006.

Lin IB, O'Sullivan PB, Coffin JA, Mak DB, Toussaint S, and Straker LM. "Disabling Chronic Low Back Pain as an Iatrogenic Disorder: A Qualitative Study in Aboriginal Australians." *BMJ Open* 3 (4) (2013): e002654. doi:10.1136/bmjopen-2013-002654.

Sandal LF, Bach K, Øverås CK, et al. "Effectiveness of App-Delivered, Tailored Self-Management Support for Adults with Lower Back Pain-Related Disability: A selfBACK Randomized Clinical Trial." *JAMA Internal Medicine* 181 (10) (2021): 1288–96. doi:10.1001/jamainternmed.2021.4097.

Stilwell P and Harman K. "An Enactive Approach to Pain: Beyond the Biopsychosocial Model." *Phenomenology and the Cognitive Sciences* 18 (4) (2019): 637–65. doi:10.1007/s11097-019-09624-7.

Waddell G. "Biopsychosocial Analysis of Low Back Pain." *Baillière's Clinical Rheumatology* 6 (3) (1992): 523–5=57. doi:10.1016/s0950-3579 (05)80126-8.

Chapter 4

Brinjikji W, Luetmer PH, Comstock B, et al. "Systematic Literature Review of Imaging Features of Spinal Degeneration in Asymptomatic Populations." *American Journal of Neuroradiology* 36 (4) (2015): 811–16. doi:10.3174/ajnr.A4173.

Christe G, Nzamba J, Desarzens L, Leuba A, Darlow B, and Pichonnaz C. "Physiotherapists' Attitudes and Beliefs About Low Back Pain Influence Their Clinical Decisions and Advice." *Musculoskeletal Science & Practice* 53 (2021): 102382. doi:10.1016/j.msksp.2021.102382.

Darlow B, Dean S, Perry M, Mathieson F, Baxter GD, and Dowell A. Easy to Harm, Hard to Heal: Patient Views About the Back. *Spine* 40 (11) (2015): 842–50. doi:10.1097/BRS.0000000000000901.

Darlow B, Dowell A, Baxter GD, Mathieson F, Perry M, and Dean S. "The Enduring Impact of What Clinicians Say to People With Low Back Pain." *Annals of Family Medicine* 11 (6) (2013): 527–34. doi:10.1370/afm.1518.

Goertz C. "Five Things Patients with Low Back Pain Need from Their Doctors—Insights from the 'Spine Squad.'" MedPage Today, March 10, 2025. https://www.medpagetoday.com/opinion/second-opinions/114573.

Melzack R and Katz J. "Pain." *Wiley Interdisciplinary Reviews: Cognitive Science* 4 (1) (2013): 1–15. doi:10.1002/wcs.1201.

Melzack R and Wall PD. "Pain Mechanisms: A New Theory." *Science* 150 (3699) (1965): 971–79. doi:10.1126/science.150.3699.971.

Stochkendahl MJ, Kjaer P, Hartvigsen J, et al. "National Clinical Guidelines for Non-Surgical Treatment of Patients with Recent Onset Low Back Pain or Lumbar Radiculopathy." *European Spine Journal* 27 (1) (2018): 60–75. doi:10.1007/s00586-017-5099-2.

Wall PD and McMahon SB. "The Relationship of Perceived Pain to Afferent Nerve Impulses." *Trends in Neurosciences* 9 (6) (1986): 254–55. doi:10.1016/0166-2236(86)90070-6.

Chapter 5

Blyth FM, Briggs AM, Schneider CH, Hoy DG, and March LM. "The Global Burden of Musculoskeletal Pain—Where to from Here?" *American Journal of Public Health* 109 (1) (2019): 35–40. doi:10.2105/AJPH.2018.304747.

Bokhour BG, Haun JN, Hyde J, Charns M, and Kligler B. "Transforming the Veterans Affairs to a Whole Health System of Care: Time for Action and Research." *Medical Care* 58 (4) (2020): 295–300. doi:10.1097/MLR.0000000000001316.

Braveman P and Gottlieb L. "The Social Determinants of Health: It's Time to Consider the Causes of the Causes." *Public Health Reports* 129 (Suppl 2) (2014): 19–31.

Campbell LC, Clauw DJ, and Keefe FJ. "Persistent Pain and Depression: A Biopsychosocial Perspective." *Biological Psychiatry* 54 (3) (2003): 399–409. doi:10.1016/s0006-3223 (03)00545-6.

de Raaij EJ, Ostelo RW, Maissan F, Mollema J, and Wittink H. "The Association of Illness Perception and Prognosis for Pain and Physical Function in Patients with Noncancer Musculoskeletal Pain:

A Systematic Literature Review." *Journal of Orthopaedic & Sports Physical Therapy* 48 (10) (2018): 789–800. doi:10.2519/jospt.2018.8072.

Kamper SJ, Apeldoorn AT, Chiarotto A, et al. "Multidisciplinary Biopsychosocial Rehabilitation for Chronic Low Back Pain: Cochrane Systematic Review and Meta-Analysis." *BMJ* 350 (2015): h444. doi:10.1136/bmj.h444.

Karran EL, Grant AR, and Moseley GL. "Low Back Pain and the Social Determinants of Health : A Systematic Review and Narrative Synthesis." *Pain* 161 (11) (2020): 2476–93. doi:10.1097/j.pain.0000000000001944.

Krejci LP, Carter K, and Gaudet T. "Whole Health: The Vision and Implementation of Personalized, Proactive, Patient-Driven Health Care for Veterans." *Medical Care* 52 (2014): S5. doi:10.1097/MLR.0000000000000226.

Waddell G. "Biopsychosocial Analysis of Low Back Pain." *Baillière's Clinical Rheumatology* 6 (3) (1992): 523–557. doi:10.1016/s0950-3579(05)80126-8.

"Whole Person Health: What You Need to Know." NCCIH. Accessed July 13, 2021. https://www.nccih.nih.gov/health/whole-person-health-what-you-need-to-know.

Chapter 6

Alzahrani H, Mackey M, Stamatakis E, Zadro JR, and Shirley D. "The Association Between Physical Activity and Low Back Pain: A Systematic Review and Meta-Analysis of Observational Studies." *Scientific Reports* 9 (1) (2019): 8244. doi:10.1038/s41598-019-44664-8.

Anheyer D, Haller H, Barth J, Lauche R, Dobos G, and Cramer H. "Mindfulness-Based Stress Reduction for Treating Low Back Pain: A Systematic Review and Meta-Analysis." *Annals of Internal Medicine* 166 (11) (2017): 799–807. doi:10.7326/M16-1997.

Bohman T, Alfredsson L, Hallqvist J, Vingård E, and Skillgate E. "The Influence of Self-Reported Leisure Time Physical Activity and the Body Mass Index on Recovery from Persistent Back Pain Among Men and Women: A Population-Based Cohort Study." *BMC Public Health* 13 (1) (2013): 385. doi:10.1186/1471-2458-13-385.

Ditre JW and Brandon TH. "Pain as a Motivator of Smoking: Effects of Pain Induction on Smoking Urge and Behavior." *Journal of Abnormal Psychology* 117 (2):467–472. doi:10.1037/0021-843X.117.2.467.

Goldthorpe J, Peters S, Lovell K, McGowan L, and Aggarwal V. "'I Just Wanted Someone to Tell Me It Wasn't All in My Mind and Do Something for Me': Qualitative Exploration of Acceptability of a CBT Based Intervention to Manage Chronic Orofacial Pain." *British Dental Journal* 220 (9) (2016): 459–63. doi:10.1038/sj.bdj.2016.332.

Hahn EJ, Rayens MK, Kirsh KL, and Passik SD. "Brief Report: Pain and Readiness to Quit Smoking Cigarettes." *Nicotine & Tobacco Research* 8 (3) (2006):473–80. doi:10.1080/14622200600670355.

Hartvigsen J, Hancock MJ, Kongsted A, et al. "What Low Back Pain Is and Why We Need to Pay Attention." *Lancet* 391 (10137) (2018): 2356–67. doi:10.1016/S0140-6736(18)30480-X.

Hayden JA, Ogilvie R, Kashif S, et al. "Exercise Treatments for Chronic Low Back Pain: A Network Meta-Analysis." *Cochrane Database of Systematic Reviews* (6) (2023). doi:10.1002/14651858.CD015608.

Hooten WM, Townsend CO, Hays JT, et al. "A Cognitive Behavioral Smoking Abstinence Intervention for Adults with Chronic Pain: A Randomized Controlled Pilot Trial." *Addictive Behaviors* 39 (3) (2014): 593–99. doi:10.1016/j.addbeh.2013.11.010.

Kamper SJ, Apeldoorn AT, Chiarotto A, et al. "Multidisciplinary Biopsychosocial Rehabilitation for Chronic Low Back Pain: Cochrane Systematic Review and Meta-Analysis." *BMJ* 350 (2015): h444. doi:10.1136/bmj.h444.

Kapos FP, Burke CA, and Goode AP. "Perceived Community Control in Adults with Acute Low Back Pain: A Community-Based Study." *International Journal of Environmental Research and Public Health* 21 (10) (2024): 1310. doi:10.3390/ijerph21101310.

Karran EL, Grant AR, and Moseley GL. "Low Back Pain and the Social Determinants of Health: A Systematic Review and Narrative Synthesis." *Pain* 161 (11) (2020): 2476–93. doi:10.1097/j.pain.0000000000001944.

Khan JS, Hah JM, and Mackey SC. "Effects of Smoking on Patients with Chronic Pain: A Propensity-Weighted Analysis on the Collaborative Health Outcomes Information Registry." *Pain* 160 (10) (2019): 2374–79. doi:10.1097/j.pain.0000000000001631.

Krejci LP, Carter K, and Gaudet T. "Whole Health: The Vision and Implementation of Personalized, Proactive, Patient-Driven Health Care for Veterans." *Medical Care* 52 (2014): S5. doi:10.1097/MLR.0000000000000226.

Li W, Lai K, Chopra N, Zheng Z, Das A, and Diwan AD. "Gut-Disc Axis: A Cause of Intervertebral Disc Degeneration and Low Back Pain?" *European Spine Journal* 31 (4) (April 2022): 917–25. doi:10.1007/s00586-022-07152-8. Epub: March 14, 2022. PMID: 35286474.

Rajasekaran S, Vasudevan G, Tangavel C, et al. "Does the Gut Microbiome Influence Disc Health and Disease? The Interplay Between Dysbiosis, Pathobionts, and Disc Inflammation: A Pilot Study." *Spine Journal* 24 (10) (October 2024): 1952–63. doi:10.1016/j.spinee.2024.06.020. Epub: June 24, 2024. PMID: 38925301.

Sun Y, Li Z, Duan J, et al. "Unveiling the Gut-Disc Axis: How Microbiome Dysbiosis Accelerates Intervertebral Disc Degeneration." *Journal of Inflammation Research* 17 (November 5, 2024): 8271–80. doi:10.2147/JIR.S487936. PMID: 39525319. PMCID: PMC11549883.

Xu HR, Zhang YH, Ngo TL, Yang QH, Du SH, and Wang XQ. "Association between smoking and Incident Back Pain: A Prospective Cohort Study with 438,510 Participants." *Journal of Global Health* 13 (2023): 04152. doi:10.7189/jogh.13.04152.

Chapter 7

Bair MJ, Matthias MS, Nyland KA, et al. "Barriers and Facilitators to Chronic Pain Self-Management: A Qualitative Study of Primary Care Patients with Comorbid Musculoskeletal Pain and Depression." *Pain Medicine* (Malden, MA) 10 (7) (2009): 1280–90. doi:10.1111/j.1526-4637.2009.00707.x.

Barlow J, Wright C, Sheasby J, Turner A, and Hainsworth J. "Self-Management Approaches for People with Chronic Conditions: A Review." *Patient Education and Counseling* 48 (2) (2002): 177–87. doi:10.1016/S0738-3991(02)00032-0.

Bourke MJ, Ferguson D, and Cooke M. "Patient Experiences of Self-Management for Chronic Low Back Pain: A Qualitative Study." *Physical Therapy & Rehabilitation Journal*. Published online March 30, 2022: pzac030. doi:10.1093/ptj/pzac030.

Caiata Zufferey M and Schulz PJ. "Self-Management of Chronic Low Back Pain: An Exploration of the Impact of a Patient-Centered Website." *Patient Education and Counseling* 77 (1) (2009): 27–32. doi:10.1016/j.pec.2009.01.016.

Devan H, Hale L, Hempel D, Saipe B, and Perry MA. "What Works and Does Not Work in a Self-Management Intervention for People with Chronic Pain? Qualitative Systematic Review and Meta-Synthesis." *Physical Therapy & Rehabilitation Journal* 98 (5) (2018): 381–97. doi:10.1093/ptj/pzy029.

Du S, Hu L, Dong J, et al. "Self-Management Program for Chronic Low Back Pain: A Systematic Review and Meta-Analysis." *Patient Education and Counseling* 100 (1) (2017): 37–49. doi:10.1016/j.pec.2016.07.029.

Haas M, Boiché J, Chevance G, et al. "Motivation Toward Physical Activity in Patients with Chronic Musculoskeletal Disorders: A Meta-Analysis of the Efficacy of Behavioural Interventions." *Scientific Reports* 14 (1) (2024): 18740. doi:10.1038/s41598-024-67948-0.

Haas M, Groupp E, Muench J, et al. "Chronic Disease Self-Management Program for Low Back Pain in the Elderly." *Journal of Manipulative and Physiological Therapeutics* 28 (4) (2005): 228–37. doi:10.1016/j.jmpt.2005.03.010.

Johnston V, Jull G, Sheppard DM, and Ellis N. "Applying Principles of Self-Management to Facilitate Workers to Return to or Remain at Work with a Chronic Musculoskeletal Condition." *Manual Therapy* 18 (4) (2013): 274–80. doi:10.1016/j.math.2013.04.001.

Kjaer P, Kongsted A, Ris I, et al. "GLA:D® Back Group-Based Patient Education Integrated with Exercises to Support Self-Management of Back Pain—Development, Theories and Scientific Evidence." *BMC Musculoskeletal Disorders* 19 (1) (2018): 418. doi:10.1186/s12891-018-2334-x.

Kongsted A, Ris I, Kjaer P, and Hartvigsen J. "Self-Management at the Core of Back Pain Care: 10 Key Points for Clinicians." *Brazilian Journal of Physical Therapy* 25 (4) (2021): 396–406. doi:10.1016/j.bjpt.2021.05.002.

Roberts KE, Beckenkamp PR, Ferreira ML, et al. "Positive Lifestyle Behaviours and Emotional Health Factors Are Associated with Low Back Pain Resilience." *European Spine Journal* 31 (12) (2022): 3616–26. doi:10.1007/s00586-022-07404-7.

Sandal LF, Bach K, Øverås CK, et al. "Effectiveness of App-Delivered, Tailored Self-Management Support for Adults with Lower Back Pain–Related Disability: A selfBACK Randomized Clinical Trial." *JAMA Internal Medicine* 181 (10) (2021): 1288–96. doi:10.1001/jamainternmed.2021.4097.

Chapter 8

Alnawwar MA, Alraddadi MI, Algethmi RA, Salem GA, Salem MA, and Alharbi AA. "The Effect of Physical Activity on Sleep Quality and Sleep Disorder: A Systematic Review." *Cureus* 15 (8) (2023): e43595. doi:10.7759/cureus.43595.

Basso JC and Suzuki WA. "The Effects of Acute Exercise on Mood, Cognition, Neurophysiology, and Neurochemical Pathways: A Review." *Brain Plasticity* 2 (2) (2017): 127–52. doi:10.3233/BPL-160040.

Beavers KM, Brinkley TE, and Nicklas BJ. "Effect of Exercise Training on Chronic Inflammation. *Clinica Chimica Acta* 411 (11–12) (2010): 785–93. doi:10.1016/j.cca.2010.02.069.

Caspersen CJ, Powell KE, and Christenson GM. "Physical Activity, Exercise, and Physical Fitness: Definitions and Distinctions for Health-Related Research." *Public Health Reports* 100 (2) (1985): 126–31.

Chastin SFM, Abaraogu U, Bourgois JG, et al. "Effects of Regular Physical Activity on the Immune System, Vaccination and Risk of Community-Acquired Infectious Disease in the General Population: Systematic Review and Meta-Analysis." *Sports Medicine* 51 (8) (2021): 1673–86. doi:10.1007/s40279-021-01466-1.

Cheung K, Hume P, and Maxwell L. "Delayed Onset Muscle Soreness : Treatment Strategies and Performance Factors." *Sports Medicine* 33 (2) (2003): 145–64. doi:10.2165/00007256-200333020-00005.

Dailey DL, Vance CGT, Rakel BA, et al. "Transcutaneous Electrical Nerve Stimulation Reduces Movement-Evoked Pain and Fatigue: A Randomized, Controlled Trial." *Arthritis & Rheumatology* 72 (5) (May 2020): 824–36. doi:10.1002/art.41170. Epub: March 18, 2020. PMID: 31738014. PMCID: PMC7188591.

Dhuli K, Naureen Z, Medori MC, et al. "Physical Activity for Health." *Journal of Preventive Medicine and Hygiene* 63 (2 Suppl 3) (2022): E150–E159. doi:10.15167/2421-4248/jpmh2022.63.2S3.2756.

Docherty S, Harley R, McAuley JJ, et al. "The Effect of Exercise on Cytokines: Implications for Musculoskeletal Health: A Narrative Review." *BMC Sports Science, Medicine and Rehabilitation* 14 (1) (2022): 5. doi:10.1186/s13102-022-00397-2.

Geneen LJ, Moore RA, Clarke C, Martin D, Colvin LA, and Smith BH. "Physical Activity and Exercise for Chronic Pain in Adults: An Overview of Cochrane Reviews." *Cochrane Database of Systematic Reviews* (1) (2017): CD011279. doi:10.1002/14651858.CD011279.pub2.

Hartvigsen J, Morsø L, Bendix T, and Manniche C. "Supervised and Non-Supervised Nordic Walking in the Treatment of Chronic Low Back Pain: A Single Blind Randomized Clinical Trial. *BMC Musculoskeletal Disorders* 11 (2010): 30. doi:10.1186/1471-2474-11-30.

Hayden JA, Ellis J, Ogilvie R, Malmivaara A, and Tulder MW van. "Exercise Therapy for Chronic Low Back Pain." *Cochrane Database of Systematic Reviews* (9) (2021). doi:10.1002/14651858.CD009790.pub2.

Hayden JA, Ogilvie R, Kashif S, et al. "Exercise Treatments for Chronic Low Back Pain: A Network Meta-Analysis." *Cochrane Database of Systematic Reviews* (6) (2023). doi:10.1002/14651858.CD015608.

Hayden JA, van Tulder MW, Malmivaara A, and Koes BW. "Exercise Therapy for Treatment of Non-Specific Low Back Pain." *Cochrane Database of Systematic Reviews* (3) (2005): CD000335. doi:10.1002/14651858.CD000335.pub2.

Irwin ML, Cartmel B, Harrigan M, et al. "Effect of the LIVESTRONG at the YMCA Exercise Program on Physical Activity, Fitness, Quality of Life, and Fatigue in Cancer Survivors." *Cancer* 123 (7) (2017): 1249–58. doi:10.1002/cncr.30456.

Kapoor G, Chauhan P, Singh G, Malhotra N, and Chahal A. "Physical Activity for Health and Fitness: Past, Present and Future." *Journal of Lifestyle Medicine* 12 (1) (2022): 9–14. doi:10.15280/jlm.2022.12.1.9.

Kent JA and Hayes KL. "Exercise Physiology from 1980 to 2020: Application of the Natural Sciences." *Kinesiology Review* 10 (3) (2021): 238–47. doi:10.1123/kr.2021-0024.

Lachman ME, Lipsitz L, Lubben J, Castaneda-Sceppa C, and Jette AM. "When Adults Don't Exercise: Behavioral Strategies to Increase Physical Activity in Sedentary Middle-Aged and Older Adults." *Innovation in Aging* 2 (1) (2018): igy007. doi:10.1093/geroni/igy007.

Lang AE, Hendrick PA, Clay L, et al. "A Randomized Controlled Trial Investigating Effects of an Individualized Pedometer Driven Walking Program on Chronic Low Back Pain." *BMC Musculoskeletal Disorders* 22 (2021). doi:10.1186/s12891-021-04060-8.

Leeuw M, Goossens MEJB, Linton SJ, Crombez G, Boersma K, and Vlaeyen JWS. The Fear-Avoidance Model of Musculoskeletal Pain: Current State of Scientific Evidence." *Journal of Behavioral Medicine* 30 (1) (2007): 77–94. doi:10.1007/s10865-006-9085-0.

Mahindru A, Patil P, and Agrawal V. "Role of Physical Activity on Mental Health and Well-Being: A Review." *Cureus* 15 (1) (2023): e33475. doi:10.7759/cureus.33475.

Nieman DC and Wentz LM. "The Compelling Link Between Physical Activity and the Body's Defense System." *Journal of Sport and Health Science* 8 (3) (2019): 201–17. doi:10.1016/j.jshs.2018.09.009.

Nystoriak MA and Bhatnagar A. "Cardiovascular Effects and Benefits of Exercise." *Frontiers in Cardiovascular Medicine* 5 (2018): 135. doi:10.3389/fcvm.2018.00135.

O'Keeffe M, O'Sullivan P, Purtill H, Bargary N, and O'Sullivan K. "Cognitive Functional Therapy Compared with a Group-Based Exercise and Education Intervention for Chronic Low Back Pain: A Multicentre Randomised Controlled Trial (RCT)." *British Journal of Sports Medicine* 54 (13) (2020): 782–89. doi:10.1136/bjsports-2019-100780.

Ruegsegger GN and Booth FW. "Health Benefits of Exercise." *Cold Spring Harbor Perspectives in Medicine* 8 (7) (2018): a029694. doi:10.1101/cshperspect.a029694.

Sluka KA, Frey-Law L, and Hoeger Bement M. "Exercise-Induced Pain and Analgesia? Underlying Mechanisms and Clinical Translation." *Pain* 159 (Suppl 1) (2018): S91–S97. doi:10.1097/j.pain.0000000000001235.

Thorén P, Floras JS, Hoffmann P, and Seals DR. "Endorphins and Exercise: Physiological Mechanisms and Clinical Implications." *Medicine & Science in Sports & Exercise* 22 (4) (1990): 417–28.

Tomoto T, Verma A, Kostroske K, et al. "One-Year Aerobic Exercise Increases Cerebral Blood Flow in Cognitively Normal Older Adults." *Journal of Cerebral Blood Flow & Metabolism* 43 (3) (2023): 404–18. doi:10.1177/0271678X221133861.

Toomey E, Currie-Murphy L, Matthews J, and Hurley DA. "The Effectiveness of Physiotherapist-Delivered Group Education and Exercise Interventions to Promote Self-Management for People with Osteoarthritis and Chronic Low Back Pain: A Rapid Review Part I. *Manual Therapy* 20 (2) (2015): 265–86. doi:10.1016/j.math.2014.10.013.

Vanti C, Andreatta S, Borghi S, Guccione AA, Pillastrini P, and Bertozzi L. "The Effectiveness of Walking Versus Exercise on Pain and Function in Chronic Low Back Pain: A Systematic Review and Meta-Analysis of Randomized Trials." *Disability and Rehabilitation* 41 (6) (2019): 622–32. doi: 10.1080/09638288.2017.1410730.

Withall J, Jago R, and Fox KR. "Why Some Do but Most Don't. Barriers and Enablers to Engaging Low-Income Groups in Physical Activity Programmes: A Mixed Methods Study." *BMC Public Health* 11 (2011): 507. doi:10.1186/1471-2458-11-507.

Wun A, Kollias P, Jeong H, et al. "Why Is Exercise Prescribed for People with Chronic Low Back Pain? A Review of the Mechanisms of Benefit Proposed by Clinical Trialists. *Musculoskeletal Science & Practice* 51(2021):102307. doi:10.1016/j.msksp.2020.102307.

Chapter 9

Anheyer D, Haller H, Lauche R, Dobos G, and Cramer H. "Yoga for Treating Low Back Pain: A Systematic Review and Meta-Analysis." *Pain* 163 (4) (2022) :e504–e517. doi:10.1097/j.pain.0000000000002416.

Chang DG, Holt JA, Sklar M, and Groessl EJ. "Yoga as a Treatment for Chronic Low Back Pain: A systematic Review of the Literature." *Journal of Orthopedics & Rheumatology* 3 (1) (January 1, 2016): 1–8. PMID: 27231715. PMCID: PMC4878447.

Hayden JA, Ogilvie R, Kashif S, et al. "Exercise Treatments for Chronic Low Back Pain: A Network Meta Analysis." *Cochrane Database of Systematic Reviews* (6) (2023). doi:10.1002/14651858.CD015608.

Nikolis A, Nikolis L, and Meron A. "Yoga as an Adjunctive Treatment for Chronic Low Back Pain: A Narrative Review." *Pain Physician* 27 (7) (2024): E661–E675.

Sherman KJ, Cherkin DC, Wellman RD, et al. "A Randomized Trial Comparing Yoga, Stretching, and a Self-Care Book for Chronic Low Back Pain." *Archives of Internal Medicine* 171 (22) (2011): 2019–26. doi:10.1001/archinternmed.2011.524.

Tankha H, Gaskins D, Shallcross A, et al. "Effectiveness of Virtual Yoga for Chronic Low Back Pain: A Randomized Clinical Trial." *JAMA Network Open* 7 (11) (2024): e2442339. doi:10.1001/jamanetworkopen.2024.42339.

Wieland LS, Skoetz N, Pilkington K, Harbin S, Vempati R, and Berman BM. "Yoga for Chronic Non-Specific Low Back Pain." *Cochrane Database of Systematic Reviews* 11 (11) (2022): CD010671. doi:10.1002/14651858.CD010671.pub3.

Chapter 10

Cheung K, Hume P, and Maxwell L. "Delayed Onset Muscle Soreness: Treatment Strategies and Performance Factors." *Sports Medicine* 33 (2) (2003): 145–64. doi:10.2165/00007256-200333020-00005.

Fernández-Rodríguez R, Álvarez-Bueno C, Cavero-Redondo I, et al. "Best Exercise Options for Reducing Pain and Disability in Adults with Chronic Low Back Pain: Pilates, Strength, Core-Based, and Mind-Body. A Network Meta-Analysis." *Journal of Orthopaedic & Sports Physical Therapy* 52 (8) (2022): 505–21. doi:10.2519/jospt.2022.10671.

Gjestvang C, Abrahamsen F, Stensrud T, and Haakstad LAH. "Motives and Barriers to Initiation and Sustained Exercise Adherence in a Fitness Club Setting—a One-Year Follow-Up Study." *Scandinavian Journal of Medicine & Science in Sports* 30 (9) (2020): 1796–1805. doi:10.1111/sms.13736.

Hayden JA, Ogilvie R, Kashif S, et al. "Exercise Treatments for Chronic Low Back Pain: A Network Meta-Analysis." *Cochrane Database of Systematic Reviews* (6) (2023). doi:10.1002/14651858.CD015608.

Lee JS and Kang SJ. "The Effects of Strength Exercise and Walking on Lumbar Function, Pain Level, and Body Composition in Chronic Back Pain Patients." *Journal of Exercise Rehabilitation* 12 (5) (October 31, 2016): 463–4=70. doi:10.12965/jer.1632650.325. PMID: 27807526, PMCID: PMC5091063.

Shiri R, Coggon D, and Falah-Hassani K. "Exercise for the Prevention of Low Back Pain: Systematic Review and Meta-Analysis of Controlled Trials." *American Journal of Epidemiology* 187 (5) (2018): 1093–1101. doi:10.1093/aje/kwx337.

Wang X, Song WJ, Ruan Y, et al. "Core Muscle Functional Strength Training for Reducing the Risk of Low Back Pain in Military Recruits: An Open-Label Randomized Controlled Trial." *Journal of Integrative Medicine* 20 (2) (2022): 145–52. doi:10.1016/j.joim.2021.12.002.

Chapter 11

Abdel Shaheed C, Ferreira GE, Dmitritchenko A, et al. "The Efficacy and Safety of Paracetamol for Pain Relief: An Overview of Systematic Reviews." *Medical Journal of Australia* 214 (7) (2021): 324–31. doi:10.5694/mja2.50992.

Annaswamy TM, Cunniff KJ, Kroll M, et al. "Lumbar Bracing for Chronic Low Back Pain: A Randomized Controlled Trial." *American Journal of Physical Medicine & Rehabilitation* 100 (8) (2021): 742–49. doi:10.1097/PHM.0000000000001743.

Arienti C, Lazzarini SG, Zaina F, et al. "Lumbar Braces and Other Assistive Devices for Treatment of Chronic Low Back Pain." *Cochrane Database of Systematic Reviews* 7 (7) (2024): CD015492. doi:10.1002/14651858.CD015492.

Barłowska-Trybulec M, Zawojska K, Szklarczyk J, and Góralska M. "Effect of Whole Body Cryotherapy on Low Back Pain and Release of Endorphins and Stress Hormones in Patients with Lumbar Spine Osteoarthritis." *Reumatologia* 60 (4) (2022): 247–51. doi:10.5114/reum.2022.119040.

Binny J, Joshua Wong NL, Garga S, et al. "Transcutaneous Electric Nerve Stimulation (TENS) for Acute Low Back Pain: Systematic Review." *Scandinavian Journal of Pain* 19 (2) (2019): 225–33. doi:10.1515/sjpain-2018-0124.

Cambron JA, Dexheimer JM, Duarte M, and Freels S. "Shoe Orthotics for the Treatment of Chronic Low Back Pain: A Randomized Controlled Trial." *Archives of Physical Medicine and Rehabilitation* 98 (9) (2017): 1752–62. doi:10.1016/j.apmr.2017.03.028.

Driessen MT, Proper KI, van Tulder MW, Anema JR, Bongers PM, and van der Beek AJ. "The Effectiveness of Physical and Organisational Ergonomic Interventions on Low Back Pain and Neck Pain: A Systematic Review." *Occupational and Environmental Medicine* 67 (4) (2010): 277–85. doi:10.1136/oem.2009.047548.

Ferreira ML, Herbert RD, Ferreira PH, et al. "The Smallest Worthwhile Effect of Nonsteroidal Anti-Inflammatory Drugs and Physiotherapy for Chronic Low Back Pain: A Benefit-Harm Trade-Off Study." *Journal of Clinical Epidemiology* 66 (12) (2013): 1397–1404. doi:10.1016/j .jclinepi.2013.02.018.

Freiwald J, Magni A, Fanlo-Mazas P, et al. "A Role for Superficial Heat Therapy in the Management of Non-Specific, Mild-to-Moderate Low Back Pain in Current Clinical Practice: A Narrative Review." *Life* 11 (8) (2021): 780. doi:10.3390/life11080780.

French SD, Cameron M, Walker BF, Reggars JW, and Esterman AJ. "Superficial Heat or Cold for Low Back Pain." *Cochrane Database of Systematic Reviews* (1) (2006): CD004750 . doi:10.1002/14651858.CD004750.pub2.

Frerick H, Keitel W, Kuhn U, Schmidt S, Bredehorst A, and Kuhlmann M. "Topical Treatment of Chronic Low Back Pain with a Capsicum Plaster." *Pain* 106 (1–2) (2003): 59–64. doi:10.1016 /s0304-3959 (03)00278-1.

Gimbel J, Linn R, Hale M, and Nicholson B. "Lidocaine Patch Treatment in Patients with Low Back Pain: Results of an Open-Label, Nonrandomized Pilot Study." *American Journal of Therapeutics* 12 (4) (2005): 311–19. doi:10.1097/01.mjt.0000164828.57392.ba.

Hines R, Keaney D, Moskowitz MH, and Prakken S. "Use of Lidocaine Patch 5% for Chronic Low Back Pain: A Report of Four Cases." *Pain Medicine* (Malden, MA) 3 (4) (2002): 361–65. doi:10.1046/j.1526-4637.2002.02051.x.

Jaromi M, Nemeth A, Kranicz J, Laczko T, and Betlehem J. "Treatment and Ergonomics Training of Work-Related Lower Back Pain and Body Posture Problems for Nurses." *Journal of Clinical Nursing* 21 (11–12) (2012): 1776–84. doi:10.1111/j.1365-2702.2012.04089.x.

Khadilkar A, Odebiyi DO, Brosseau L, and Wells GA. "Transcutaneous Electrical Nerve Stimulation (TENS) Versus Placebo for Chronic Low Back Pain." *Cochrane Database of Systematic Reviews* (4) (2008): CD003008. doi:10.1002/14651858.CD003008.pub3.

Kong L, Zhou X, Huang Q, et al. "The Effects of Shoes and Insoles for Low Back Pain: A Systematic Review and Meta-Analysis of Randomized Controlled Trials." *Research in Sports Medicine* 28 (4) (2020): 572–87. doi:10.1080/15438627.2020.1798238.

Leemans L, Elma Ö, Nijs J, et al. "Transcutaneous Electrical Nerve Stimulation and Heat to Reduce Pain in a Chronic Low Back Pain Population: A Randomized Controlled Clinical Trial. *Brazilian Journal of Physical Therapy* 25 (1) (2021): 86–96. doi:10.1016/j.bjpt.2020.04.001.

Machado GC, Maher CG, Ferreira PH, Day RO, Pinheiro MB, and Ferreira ML. "Non-Steroidal Anti-Inflammatory Drugs for Spinal Pain: A Systematic Review and Meta-Analysis." *Annals of the Rheumatic Diseases* 76 (7) (2017): 1269–78. doi:10.1136/annrheumdis-2016-210597.

Malanga GA, Yan N, and Stark J. "Mechanisms and Efficacy of Heat and Cold Therapies for Musculoskeletal Injury." *Postgraduate Medicine* 127 (1) (2015): 57–65. doi:10.1080/00325481.2015.992719.

Malmivaara A, Häkkinen U, Aro T, et al. "The Treatment of Acute Low Back Pain—Bed Rest, Exercises, or Ordinary Activity?" *New England Journal of Medicine* 332 (6) (1995): 351–55. doi:10.1056/NEJM199502093320602.

Mattila VM, Sillanpää P, Salo T, Laine HJ, Mäenpää H, and Pihlajamäki H. "Orthotic Insoles Do Not Prevent Physical Stress–Induced Low Back Pain." *European Spine Journal* 20 (1) (2011): 100–104. doi:10.1007/s00586-010-1496-5.

Migliorini F, Maffulli N, Eschweiler J, Tingart M, and Baroncini A. "Non-Steroidal Anti-Inflammatory Drugs and Gabapentinoids for Chronic Lumbar Pain: A Bayesian Network Meta-Analysis of Randomized Controlled Trials." *British Medical Bulletin* 138 (1) (2021): 85–95. doi:10.1093/bmb/ldab003.

Milne S, Welch V, Brosseau L, et al. "Transcutaneous Electrical Nerve Stimulation (TENS) for Chronic Low Back Pain." *Cochrane Database of Systematic Reviews* (2) (2001): CD003008. doi:10.1002/14651858.CD003008.

Nadler SF, Steiner DJ, Erasala GN, et al. "Continuous Low-Level Heat Wrap Therapy Provides More Efficacy Than Ibuprofen and Acetaminophen for Acute Low Back Pain." *Spine* 27 (10) (2002): 1012–17. doi:10.1097/00007632-200205150-00003.

Oleiwi MA, Shah SZA, Bilal H, et al. "Efficacy of Orthotic Support in Mitigating Low Back Pain and Disability in Low Back Pain Sufferers." *Journal of Back and Musculoskeletal Rehabilitation* 36 (5) (2023): 1111–25. doi:10.3233/BMR-220200.

Papuga MO and Cambron J. "Foot Orthotics for Low Back Pain: The State of Our Understanding and Recommendations for Future Research." *Foot* (Edinburgh, Scotland) 26 (2016): 53–57. doi:10.1016/j.foot.2015.12.002.

Safaeian A, Shahsanai A, and Kiyany F. "Corrective Exercises or Ergonomic Principles for Workers with Low Back Pain." *Indian Journal of Occupational and Environmental Medicine* 25 (4) (2021): 204–8. doi:10.4103/ijoem.IJOEM_255_19.

Santana JA, Klass S, and Felix ER. "The Efficacy, Effectiveness and Safety of 5% Transdermal Lidocaine Patch for Chronic Low Back Pain: A Narrative Review." *PM & R* 12 (12) (2020): 1260–67. doi:10.1002/pmrj.12366.

Saragiotto BT, Machado GC, Ferreira ML, Pinheiro MB, Abdel Shaheed C, and Maher CG. "Paracetamol for Low Back Pain." *Cochrane Database of Systematic Reviews* (6) (2016): CD012230. doi:10.1002/14651858.CD012230.

Schott C, Zirke S, Schmelzle JM, Kaiser C, and Fernández LA. "Effectiveness of Lumbar Orthoses in Low Back Pain: Review of the Literature and Our Results." *Orthopedic Reviews* 10 (4) (2018): 7791. doi:10.4081/or.2018.7791.

Schreijenberg M, Chiarotto A, Mauff KAL, Lin CWC, Maher CG, and Koes BW. "Inferential Reproduction Analysis Demonstrated That 'Paracetamol for Acute Low Back Pain' Trial Conclusions Were Reproducible." *Journal of Clinical Epidemiology* 121 (2020): 45–54. doi:10.1016/j.jclinepi.2020.01.010.

Swain CTV, Pan F, Owen PJ, Schmidt H, and Belavy DL. "No Consensus on Causality of Spine Postures or Physical Exposure and Low Back Pain: A Systematic Review of Systematic Reviews." *Journal of Biomechanics*102 (2020): 109312. doi:10.1016/j.jbiomech.2019.08.006.

Tamartash H, Bahrpeyma F, and Dizaji MM. "The Effect of Transcutaneous Electrical Nerve Stimulation on Pain and Electrical Stimulation Muscle Thickness in Patients with Non-Specific Chronic Low Back Pain–Based Ultrasonographic Evaluation." *Pain Management* 13 (2) (2023): 87–94. doi:10.2217/pmt-2022-0069.

Vance CG, Dailey DL, Rakel BA, and Sluka KA. "Using TENS for Pain Control: The State of the Evidence." *Pain Management* 4 (3) (May 2014): 197–209. doi:10.2217/pmt.14.13. PMID: 24953072. PMCID: PMC4186747.

Verville L, Hincapié CA, Southerst D, et al. "Systematic Review to Inform a World Health Organization (WHO) Clinical Practice Guideline: Benefits and Harms of Transcutaneous Electrical Nerve Stimulation (TENS) for Chronic Primary Low Back Pain in Adults." *Journal of Occupational Rehabilitation* 33 (4) (2023): 651–60. doi:10.1007/s10926-023-10121-7.

Vick JS, Zimmerman J, Hicks S, Biekert A, and Abd-Elsayed A. "Efficacy of Back Bracing in Treating Chronic Low Back Pain." *Brain Sciences* 14 (11) (2024): 1100. doi:10.3390/brainsci14111100.

Voute M, Morel V, and Pickering G. "Topical Lidocaine for Chronic Pain Treatment." *Drug Design. Development and Therapy* 15(2021): 4091–103. doi:10.2147/DDDT.S328228.

Waddell G, Feder G, and Lewis M. "Systematic Reviews of Bed Rest and Advice to Stay Active for Acute Low Back Pain." *British Journal of General Practice* 47 (423) (1997): 647–52.

Chapter 12

Asano H, Plonka D, and Weeger J. "Effectiveness of Acupuncture for Nonspecific Chronic Low Back Pain: A Systematic Review and Meta-Analysis." *Medical Acupuncture* 34 (2) (2022): 96–106. doi:10.1089/acu.2021.0057.

Baroncini A, Maffulli N, Eschweiler J, Molsberger F, Klimuch A, and Migliorini F. "Acupuncture in Chronic Aspecific Low Back Pain: A Bayesian Network Meta-Analysis." *Journal of Orthopaedic Surgery* 17 (1) (2022): 319. doi:10.1186/s13018-022-03212-3.

Brinkhaus B, Witt CM, Jena S, et al. "Acupuncture in Patients with Chronic Low Back Pain: A Randomized Controlled Trial." *Archives of Internal Medicine*166 (4) (2006): 450–57. doi:10.1001/archinte.166.4.450.

Bronfort G, Haas M, Evans RL, and Bouter LM. "Efficacy of Spinal Manipulation and Mobilization for Low Back Pain and Neck Pain: A Systematic Review and Best Evidence Synthesis. *Spine Journal* 4 (3) (2004): 335–56. doi:10.1016/j.spinee.2003.06.002.

Cagnie B, Vinck E, Beernaert A, and Cambier D. "How Common Are Side Effects of Spinal Manipulation and Can These Side Effects Be Predicted?" *Manual Therapy* 9 (3) (2004): 151–56. doi:10.1016/j.math.2004.03.001.

Chu ECP, Trager RJ, Lee LYK, and Niazi IK. "A Retrospective Analysis of the Incidence of Severe Adverse Events Among Recipients of Chiropractic Spinal Manipulative Therapy." *Scientific Reports* 13 (1) (2023): 1254. doi:10.1038/s41598-023-28520-4.

Coronado RA, Gay CW, Bialosky JE, Carnaby GD, Bishop MD, and George SZ. "Changes in Pain Sensitivity Following Spinal Manipulation: A Systematic Review and Meta-Analysis." *Journal of Electromyography and Kinesiology* 22 (5) (2012): 752–67. doi:10.1016/j.jelekin.2011.12.013.

Coulter ID, Crawford C, Hurwitz EL, et al. "Manipulation and Mobilization for Treating Chronic Low Back Pain: A Systematic Review and Meta-Analysis. *Spine Journal* 18 (5) (2018): 866–79. doi:10.1016/j.spinee.2018.01.013.

DeVocht JW, Pickar JG, and Wilder DG. "Spinal Manipulation Alters Electromyographic Activity of Paraspinal Muscles: A Descriptive Study." *Journal of Manipulative and Physiological Therapeutics* 28 (7) (2005): 465–71. doi:10.1016/j.jmpt.2005.07.002.

Eklund A, Jensen I, Lohela-Karlsson M, et al. "The Nordic Maintenance Care Program: Effectiveness of Chiropractic Maintenance Care Versus Symptom-Guided Treatment for Recurrent and Persistent Low Back Pain—a Pragmatic Randomized Controlled Trial." *PloS One* 13 (9) (2018): e0203029. doi:10.1371/journal.pone.0203029.

Farley J, Taylor-Swanson L, Koppenhaver S, Thackeray A, Magel J, and Fritz JM. "The Effect of Combining Spinal Manipulation and Dry Needling in Individuals with Nonspecific Low Back Pain." *Journal of Pain* 25 (8) (2024): 104506. doi:10.1016/j.jpain.2024.03.002.

Furlan AD, Giraldo M, Baskwill A, Irvin E, and Imamura M. "Massage for Low-Back Pain." *Cochrane Database of Systematic Reviews* (9) (2015): CD001929. doi:10.1002/14651858.CD001929.pub3.

George SZ, Fritz JM, Silfies SP, et al. "Interventions for the Management of Acute and Chronic Low Back Pain: Revision 2021." *Journal of Orthopaedic & Sports Physical Therapy* 51 (11) (2021): CPG1-CPG60. doi:10.2519/jospt.2021.0304.

Hancock MJ, Maher CG, and Latimer J. "Spinal Manipulative Therapy for Acute Low Back Pain: A Clinical Perspective." *Journal of Manual & Manipulative Therapy* 16 (4) (2008): 198–203. doi:10.1179/106698108790818279.

Hanrahan S, Van Lunen BL, Tamburello M, and Walker ML. "The Short-Term Effects of Joint Mobilizations on Acute Mechanical Low Back Dysfunction in Collegiate Athletes." *Journal of Athletic Training* 40 (2) (2005):88–93.

Hu HT, Gao H, Ma RJ, Zhao XF, Tian HF, and Li L. "Is Dry Needling Effective for Low Back Pain? A Systematic Review and PRISMA-Compliant Meta-Analysis." *Medicine* (Baltimore) 97 (26) (2018): e11225. doi:10.1097/MD.0000000000011225.

Johnston V, Jull G, Sheppard DM, and Ellis N. "Applying Principles of Self-Management to Facilitate Workers to Return to or Remain at Work with a Chronic Musculoskeletal Condition." *Manual Therapy* 18 (4) (2013): 274–80. doi:10.1016/j.math.2013.04.001.

Kamali F, Panahi F, Ebrahimi S, and Abbasi L. "Comparison between massage and routine Physical Therapy in Women with Sub Acute and Chronic Nonspecific Low Back Pain." *Journal of Back and Musculoskeletal Rehabilitation* 27 (4) (2014): 475–80. doi:10.3233/BMR-140468.

Kingston J, Raggio C, Spencer K, Stalaker K, and Tuchin PJ. "A Review of the Literature on Chiropractic and Insomnia." *Journal of Chiropractic Medicine* 9 (3) (2010): 121–26. doi:10.1016/j.jcm.2010.03.003.

Koes BW, Bouter LM, van Mameren H, et al. "The Effectiveness of Manual Therapy, Physiotherapy, and Treatment by the General Practitioner for Nonspecific Back and Neck Complaints. A Randomized Clinical Trial." *Spine* 17 (1) (1992). doi:10.1097/00007632-199201000-00005.

Koppenhaver SL, Fritz JM, Hebert JJ, et al. "Association Between Changes in Abdominal and Lumbar Multifidus Muscle Thickness and Clinical Improvement After Spinal Manipulation." *Journal of Orthopaedic & Sports Physical Therapy* 41 (6) (2011): 389–99. doi:10.2519/jospt.2011.3632.

Krekoukias G, Gelalis ID, Xenakis T, Gioftsos G, Dimitriadis Z, and Sakellari V. "Spinal Mobilization vs. Conventional Physiotherapy in the Management of Chronic Low Back Pain due to Spinal Disk Degeneration: A Randomized Controlled Trial." *Journal of Manual & Manipulative Therapy* 25 (2) (2017): 66–73. doi:10.1080/10669817.2016.1184435.

Lee JH, Choi TY, Lee MS, Lee H, Shin BC, and Lee H. "Acupuncture for Acute Low Back Pain: A Systematic Review." *Clinical Journal of Pain* 29 (2) (2013):172–85. doi:10.1097/AJP.0b013e31824909f9.

"Managing Low Back Pain: Exercise, Manual Therapy, and Education." *Journal of Orthopaedic & Sports Physical Therapy* 51 (11) (2021): 535. doi:10.2519/jospt.2021.0508.

Mu J, Furlan AD, Lam WY, Hsu MY, Ning Z, and Lao L. "Acupuncture for Chronic Nonspecific Low Back Pain." *Cochrane Database of Systematic Reviews*12 (12) (2020): CD013814. doi:10.1002/14651858.CD013814.

Pickar JG. "Neurophysiological Effects of Spinal Manipulation." *Spine Journal* 2 (5) (2002): 357–71. doi:10.1016/s1529-9430 (02)00400-x.

Qaseem A, Wilt TJ, McLean RM, Forciea MA, and Clinical Guidelines Committee of the American College of Physicians. "Noninvasive Treatments for Acute, Subacute, and Chronic Low Back Pain: A Clinical Practice Guideline from the American College of Physicians." *Annals of Internal Medicine* 166 (7) (2017): 514–30. doi:10.7326/M16-2367.

Rajfur J, Rajfur K, Kosowski Ł, et al. "The Effectiveness of Dry Needling in Patients with Chronic Low Back Pain: A Prospective, Randomized, Single-Blinded Study." *Scientific Reports* 12 (1) (2022): 15803. doi:10.1038/s41598-022-19980-1.

Rubinstein SM, de Zoete A, van Middelkoop M, Assendelft WJJ, de Boer MR, and van Tulder MW. "Benefits and Harms of Spinal Manipulative Therapy for the Treatment of Chronic Low Back Pain: Systematic Review and Meta-Analysis of Randomised Controlled Trials." *BMJ* 364 (2019): l689. doi:10.1136/bmj.l689.

Thomas JS, Clark BC, Russ DW, et al. "Effect of Spinal Manipulative and Mobilization Therapies in Young Adults with Mild to Moderate Chronic Low Back Pain: A Randomized Clinical Trial." *JAMA Network Open* 3 (8) (2020): e2012589. doi:10.1001/jamanetworkopen.2020.12589.

Trager RJ, Bejarano G, Perfecto RPT, Blackwood ER, and Goertz CM. "Chiropractic and Spinal Manipulation: A Review of Research Trends, Evidence Gaps, and Guideline Recommendations." *Journal of Clinical Medicine* 13 (19) (2024): 5668. doi:10.3390/jcm13195668.

Trager RJ, Daniels CJ, Perez JA, Casselberry RM, and Dusek JA. "Association Between Chiropractic Spinal Manipulation and Lumbar Discectomy in Adults with Lumbar Disc Herniation and Radiculopathy: Retrospective Cohort Study Using United States' Data." *BMJ Open*. Published online December 1, 2022. doi:10.1136/bmjopen-2022-068262.

Wang XQ, Wang YL, Witchalls J, et al. "Physical Therapy for Acute and Sub-Acute Low Back Pain: A Systematic Review and Expert Consensus." *Clinical Rehabilitation* 38 (6) (2024): 715–31. doi:10.1177/02692155241229398.

Waqas MS, Karimi H, Ahmad A, Rafiq S, Anwar N, and Liaqat S. "The Effects of Spinal Manipulation Added to Exercise on Pain and Quality of Life in Patients with Thoracic Spinal Pain: A Randomized Controlled Trial." *BioMed Research International* (2023): 7537335. doi:10.1155/2023/7537335.

"WHO Guideline for Non-Surgical Management of Chronic Primary Low Back Pain in Adults in Primary and Community Care Settings." World Health Organization. Accessed December 15, 2023. https://www.who.int/publications-detail-redirect/9789240081789.

Chapter 13

Akmeşe ZB and Oran NT. "Effects of Progressive Muscle Relaxation Exercises Accompanied by Music on Low Back Pain and Quality of Life During Pregnancy." *Journal of Midwifery & Women's Health* 59 (5) (2014): 503–9. doi:10.1111/jmwh.12176.

Anheyer D, Haller H, Barth J, Lauche R, Dobos G, and Cramer H. "Mindfulness-Based Stress Reduction for Treating Low Back Pain: A Systematic Review and Meta-Analysis." *Annals of Internal Medicine* 166 (11) (2017): 799–807. doi:10.7326/M16-1997.

Banth S and Ardebil MD. "Effectiveness of Mindfulness Meditation on Pain and Quality of Life of Patients with Chronic Low Back Pain." *International Journal of Yoga* 8 (2) (2015): 128–33. doi:10.4103/0973-6131.158476.

Cherkin DC, Sherman KJ, Balderson BH, et al. "Effect of Mindfulness-Based Stress Reduction vs. Cognitive Behavioral Therapy or Usual Care on Back Pain and Functional Limitations in Adults with Chronic Low Back Pain: A Randomized Clinical Trial." *JAMA* 315 (12) (2016): 1240–49. doi:10.1001/jama.2016.2323.

Cramer H, Haller H, Lauche R, and Dobos G. "Mindfulness-Based Stress Reduction for Low Back Pain. A Systematic Review." *BMC Complementary & Alternative Medicine* 12 (2012): 162. doi:10.1186/1472-6882-12-162.

Garland EL, Hanley AW, Nakamura Y, et al. "Mindfulness-Oriented Recovery Enhancement vs. Supportive Group Therapy for Co-Occurring Opioid Misuse and Chronic Pain in Primary Care: A Randomized Clinical Trial." *JAMA Internal Medicine* 182 (4) (2022): 407–17. doi:10.1001/jamainternmed.2022.0033.

Lin TH, Tam KW, Yang YL, Liou TH, Hsu TH, and Rau CL. "Meditation-Based Therapy for Chronic Low Back Pain Management: A Systematic Review and Meta-Analysis of Randomized Controlled Trials." *Pain Medicine* (Malden, MA) 23 (10) (2022): 1800–811. doi:10.1093/pm/pnac037.

Manolaki S, Gkiatas I, Sioutis S, et al. "Relaxation Techniques in Low Back Pain Patients: A Randomized Controlled Trial." *Journal of Long-Term Effects of Medical Implants* 31 (2) (2021): 39–44. doi:10.1615/JLongTermEffMedImplants.2021037026.

Mehling WE, Brintz CE, Hartogensis W, et al. "Development and Initial Validation of Mindfulness-Based Pain Reduction (MBPR) in Patients with Chronic Low Back Pain." *Journal of Pain Research* 18 (2025): 785–801. doi:10.2147/JPR.S507003.

Michalsen A, Kunz N, Jeitler M, et al. "Effectiveness of Focused Meditation for Patients with Chronic Low Back Pain: A Randomized Controlled Clinical Trial." *Complementary Therapies in Medicine* 26 (2016): 79–84. doi:10.1016/j.ctim.2016.03.010.

Morone NE, Greco CM, and Weiner DK. "Mindfulness Meditation for the Treatment of Chronic Low Back Pain in Older Adults: A Randomized Controlled Pilot Study." *Pain* 134 (3) (2008): 310–19. doi:10.1016/j.pain.2007.04.038.

Niazi AK and Niazi SK. "Mindfulness-Based Stress Reduction: A Non-Pharmacological Approach for Chronic Illnesses." *North American Journal of Medicine and Science* 3 (1) (2011): 20–23. doi:10.4297/najms.2011.320.

Paschali M, Lazaridou A, Sadora J, et al. "Mindfulness-Based Interventions for Chronic Low Back Pain: A Systematic Review and Meta-Analysis." *Clinical Journal of Pain* 40 (2) (2024): 105–13. doi:10.1097/AJP.0000000000001173.

Qaseem A, Wilt TJ, McLean RM, Forciea MA, and Clinical Guidelines Committee of the American College of Physicians. "Noninvasive Treatments for Acute, Subacute, and Chronic Low Back Pain: A Clinical Practice Guideline from the American College of Physicians." *Annals of Internal Medicine* 166 (7) (2017): 514–30. doi:10.7326/M16-2367.

Schmidt H and Pilat C. "Effects of Meditation on Pain Intensity, Physical Function, Quality of Life and Depression in Adults with Low Back Pain—a Systematic Review with Meta-Analysis." *Complementary Therapies in Medicine* 72 (2023): 102924. doi:10.1016/j.ctim.2023.102924.

Vambheim SM, Kyllo TM, Hegland S, and Bystad M. "Relaxation Techniques as an Intervention for Chronic Pain: A Systematic Review of Randomized Controlled Trials." *Heliyon* 7 (8) (2021): e07837. doi:10.1016/j.heliyon.2021.e07837.

"WHO Guideline for Non-Surgical Management of Chronic Primary Low Back Pain in Adults in Primary and Community Care Settings." World Health Organization. Accessed December 15, 2023. https://www.who.int/publications-detail-redirect/9789240081789.

Chapter 14

Bunzli S, Gillham D, and Esterman A. "Physiotherapy-Provided Operant Conditioning in the Management of Low Back Pain Disability: A Systematic Review." *Physiotherapy Research International* 16 (1) (2011): 4–19. doi:10.1002/pri.465.

Darnall BD, Burns JW, Hong J, et al. "Empowered Relief, Cognitive Behavioral Therapy, and Health Education for People with Chronic Pain: A Comparison of Outcomes at 6-Month Follow-Up for a Randomized Controlled Trial." *Pain Reports* 9 (1) (2024): e1116.

Gatchel RJ and Rollings KH. "Evidence Informed Management of Chronic Low Back Pain with Cognitive Behavioral Therapy." *Spine Journal* 8 (1) (2008): 40–44. doi:10.1016/j.spinee.2007.10.007.

Groot D, van Hooff ML, Kroeze RJ, et al. "Long-Term Results of an Intensive Cognitive Behavioral Pain Management Program for Patients with Chronic Low Back Pain: A Concise Report of an Extended Cohort with a Minimum of 5-Year Follow-Up." *European Spine Journal* 28 (7) (2019): 1579–85. doi:10.1007/s00586-019-05967-6.

Hajihasani A, Rouhani M, Salavati M, Hedayati R, and Kahlaee AH. "The Influence of Cognitive Behavioral Therapy on Pain, Quality of Life, and Depression in Patients Receiving Physical Therapy for Chronic Low Back Pain: A Systematic Review." *PM & R* 11 (2) (2019): 167–76. doi:10.1016/j.pmrj.2018.09.029.

Henschke N, Ostelo RW, van Tulder MW, et al. "Behavioural Treatment for Chronic Low Back Pain." *Cochrane Database of Systematic Reviews* (7) (2010): CD002014. doi:10.1002/14651858.CD002014.pub3.

Johnson RE, Jones GT, Wiles NJ, et al."Active Exercise, Education, and Cognitive Behavioral Therapy for Persistent Disabling Low Back Pain: A Randomized Controlled Trial." *Spine* 32 (15) (2007): 1578–85. doi:10.1097/BRS.0b013e318074f890.

Nicholas MK, Wilson PH, and Goyen J. "Operant-Behavioural and Cognitive-Behavioural Treatment for Chronic Low Back Pain." *Behavior Research and Therapy*29 (3) (1991): 225–38. doi:10.1016/0005-7967(91)90112-g.

Ploesser M and Martin D. "Mechanism of Action of Mindfulness-Based Interventions for Pain Relief: A Systematic Review." *Journal of Integrative and Complementary Medicine* 30 (12) (2024): 1162–78. doi:10.1089/jicm.2023.0328.

Stilwell P and Harman K. "An Enactive Approach to Pain: Beyond the Biopsychosocial Model." *Phenomenology and Cognitive Sciences* 18 (4) (2019): 637–65. doi:10.1007/s11097-019-09624-7.

Yang J, Lo WLA, Zheng F, Cheng X, Yu Q, and Wang C. "Evaluation of Cognitive Behavioral Therapy on Improving Pain, Fear Avoidance, and Self-Efficacy in Patients with Chronic Low Back Pain: A Systematic Review and Meta-Analysis." *Pain Research and Management* (2022): 4276175. doi:10.1155/2022/4276175.

Zhang Q, Xu H, Wang Y, Jiang J, Xue Q, and Qiu Z. "Efficacy of Cognitive Behavioral Therapy for Reducing Pain Susceptibility and Increasing Social Engagement in Patients with Chronic Low Back Pain: A Systematic Review and Meta-Analysis." *Medicine* (Baltimore) 102 (45) (2023): e35269. doi:10.1097/MD.0000000000035269.

Chapter 15

Abdel Shaheed C, Maher CG, Williams KA, Day R, and McLachlan AJ. "Efficacy, Tolerability, and Dose-Dependent Effects of Opioid Analgesics for Low Back Pain: A Systematic Review and Meta-Analysis." *JAMA Internal Medicine* 176 (7) (2016): 958–68. doi:10.1001/jamainternmed.2016.1251.

Atkinson JH, Slater MA, Capparelli EV, et al. "A Randomized Controlled Trial of Gabapentin for Chronic Low Back Pain with and Without a Radiating Component." *Pain* 157 (7) (2016): 1499–1507. doi:10.1097/j.pain.0000000000000554.

Bafail D, Mohammed HE, Bady Z, Akl AZ, and Shehata MSA. "Duloxetine for Individuals with Chronic Back Pain: A Systematic Review and Meta-Analysis of Randomized Controlled Trials." *Experimental and Therapeutic Medicine* 28 (6) (2024): 448. doi:10.3892/etm.2024.12738.

Baroncini A, Maffulli N, Al-Zyoud H, Bell A, Sevic A, and Migliorini F. "Nonopioid Pharmacological Management of Acute Low Back Pain: A Level I of Evidence Systematic Review." *Journal of Orthopaedic Research* 41 (8) (2023): 1781–91. doi:10.1002/jor.25508.

Cashin AG, Folly T, Bagg MK, et al. "Efficacy, Acceptability, and Safety of Muscle Relaxants for Adults with Non-Specific Low Back Pain: Systematic Review and Meta-Analysis." *BMJ* 374 (2021): n1446. doi:10.1136/bmj.n1446.

Cashin AG, Wand BM, O'Connell NE, et al. "Pharmacological Treatments for Low Back Pain in Adults: An Overview of Cochrane Reviews." *Cochrane Database of Systematic Reviews* (4) (2023). doi:10.1002/14651858.CD013815.pub2.

Chou R, Pinto RZ, Fu R, et al. "Systemic Corticosteroids for Radicular and Non-Radicular Low Back Pain." *Cochrane Database of Systematic Reviews* (10) (2022): CD012450. doi:10.1002/14651858.CD012450.pub2.

Deyo RA, Korff MV, and Duhrkoop D. "Opioids for Low Back Pain." *BMJ* 350 (2015): g6380. doi:10.1136/bmj.g6380.

Dowell D, Ragan KR, Jones CM, et al. "CDC Clinical Practice Guideline for Prescribing Opioids for Pain—United States, 2022." *MMWR* 71 (3) (2022): 1–95. doi:10.15585/mmwr.rr7103a1.

Friedman BW, Irizarry E, Solorzano C, et al. "Diazepam Is No Better than Placebo When Added to Naproxen for Acute Low Back Pain." *Annals of Emergency Medicine* 70 (2) (2017): 169–76.e1. doi:10.1016/j.annemergmed.2016.10.002.

Goldberg H, Firtch W, Tyburski M, et al. "Oral Steroids for Acute Radiculopathy due to a Herniated Lumbar Disk." *JAMA* 313 (19) (2015):1915–23. doi:10.1001/jama.2015.4468.

Hartvigsen J, Hancock MJ, Kongsted A, et al. "What Low Back Pain Is and Why We Need to Pay Attention." *Lancet* 391 (10137) (2018): 2356–67. doi:10.1016/S0140-6736(18)30480-X.

Hoy D, Brooks P, Blyth F, and Buchbinder R. "The Epidemiology of Low Back Pain." *Best Practice & Research: Clinical Rheumatology* 24 (6) (2010): 769–81. doi:10.1016/j.berh.2010.10.002.

Hudson TJ, Edlund MJ, Steffick DE, Tripathi SP, and Sullivan MD. "Epidemiology of Regular Prescribed Opioid Use: Results from a National, Population-Based Survey." *Journal of Pain and Symptom Management* 36 (3) (2008): 280–88. doi:10.1016/j.jpainsymman.2007.10.003.

Jones CMP, Day RO, Koes BW, et al. "Opioid Analgesia for Acute Low Back Pain and Neck Pain (the OPAL Trial): A Randomised Placebo-Controlled Trial." *Lancet* 402 (10398) (2023): 304–12. doi:10.1016/S0140-6736(23)00404-X.

Maloy GC, Halperin SJ, Ratnasamy PP, and Grauer JN. "Characterizing Gabapentinoid Use Among Patients with Isolated Low Back Pain." *Global Spine Journal* 15 (2) (2025): 1106–12. doi:10.1177/21925682231224390.

Oldfield BJ, Gleeson B, Morford KL, et al. "Long-Term Use of Muscle Relaxant Medications for Chronic Pain: A Systematic Review." *JAMA Network Open* 7 (9) (2024): e2434835. doi:10.1001/jamanetworkopen.2024.34835.

Qaseem A, Wilt TJ, McLean RM, Forciea MA, and Clinical Guidelines Committee of the American College of Physicians. "Noninvasive Treatments for Acute, Subacute, and Chronic Low Back Pain: A Clinical Practice Guideline from the American College of Physicians." *Annals of Internal Medicine* 166 (7) (2017): 514–30. doi:10.7326/M16-2367.

Shanthanna H, Gilron I, Rajarathinam M, et al. "Benefits and Safety of Gabapentinoids in Chronic Low Back Pain: A Systematic Review and Meta-Analysis of Randomized Controlled Trials." *PLoS Medicine* 14 (8) (2017): e1002369. doi:10.1371/journal.pmed.1002369.

Shehata M, Mohammed HE, and Bady Z. "Efficacy and Safety of Duloxetine in Chronic Low Back Pain: A Comprehensive Systematic Review and Meta-Analysis (P5-13.001)." *Neurology* 102 (7) (Suppl 1) (2024): 6248. doi:10.1212/WNL.0000000000206345.

Shmagel A, Foley R, and Ibrahim H. "Epidemiology of Chronic Low Back Pain in US Adults: National Health and Nutrition Examination Survey, 2009–2010." *Arthritis Care & Research* 68 (11) (2016):1688–94. doi:10.1002/acr.22890.

Shmagel A, Ngo L, Ensrud K, and Foley R. "Prescription Medication Use Among Community-Based US Adults with Chronic Low Back Pain: A Cross-Sectional Population Based Study." *Journal of Pain* 19 (10) (2018): 1104–12. doi:10.1016/j.jpain.2018.04.004.

Tatit RT, Poetscher AW, and Oliveira CAC de. "Pregabalin and Gabapentin for Chronic Low Back Pain Without Radiculopathy: A Systematic Review." *Arquivos de Neuro-Psiquiatria* 81 (6) (2023): 564–76. doi:10.1055/s-0043-1764414.

Tracey I. "Getting the Pain You Expect: Mechanisms of Placebo, Nocebo and Reappraisal Effects in Humans." *Nature Medicine* 16 (11) (2010):1277–83. doi:10.1038/nm.2229.

"U.S. Overdose Deaths Involving Prescription Opioids, 1999–2023." National Institute for Drug Abuse, National Institutes of Health. https://nida.nih.gov/research-topics/trends-statistics/overdose-death-rates#Fig4.

"WHO Guideline for Non-Surgical Management of Chronic Primary Low Back Pain in Adults in Primary and Community Care Settings." World Health Organization. Accessed December 15, 2023. https://www.who.int/publications-detail-redirect/9789240081789.

Wiffen PJ, Derry S, Bell RF, et al. "Gabapentin for Chronic Neuropathic Pain in Adults." Cochrane Library. Accessed August 11, 2025. https://www.cochranelibrary.com/cdsr/doi/10.1002/14651858.CD007938.pub4/full.

Chapter 16

Busse JW, Genevay S, Agarwal A, et al. "Commonly Used Interventional Procedures for Non-Cancer Chronic Spine Pain: A Clinical Practice Guideline." *BMJ* 388 (2025): e079970. doi:10.1136/bmj-2024-079970.

Chang MC and Park D. "The Effect of Intradiscal Platelet-Rich Plasma Injection for Management of Discogenic Lower Back Pain: A Meta-Analysis." *Journal of Pain Research* 14 (2021): 505–12. doi:10.2147/JPR.S292335.

Chou R, Pinto RZ, Fu R, et al. "Systemic Corticosteroids for Radicular and Non-Radicular Low Back Pain." *Cochrane Database of Systematic Reviews* (10) (2022): CD012450. doi:10.1002/14651858.CD012450.pub2.

Curatolo M, Rundell SD, Gold LS, et al. "Long-Term Effectiveness of Epidural Steroid Injections After New Episodes of Low Back Pain in Older Adults." *European Journal of Pain*. Published online May 23, 2022. doi:10.1002/ejp.1975.

Dagenais S, Yelland MJ, Del Mar C, and Schoene ML. "Prolotherapy Injections for Chronic Low Back Pain." *Cochrane Database of Systematic Reviews* (2) (2007): CD004059. doi:10.1002/14651858.CD004059.pub3.

Eworuke E, Crisafi L, Liao J, et al. "Risk of Serious Spinal Adverse Events Associated with Epidural Corticosteroid Injections in the Medicare Population." *Regional Anesthesia & Pain Medicine* 46 (3) (2021): 203–09. doi:10.1136/rapm-2020-101778.

Maas ET, Ostelo RWJG, Niemisto L, et al. "Radiofrequency Denervation for Chronic Low Back Pain." *Cochrane Database of Systematic Reviews* (10) (2015): CD008572. doi:10.1002/14651858.CD008572.pub2.

Oliveira CB, Maher CG, Ferreira ML, et al. "Epidural Corticosteroid Injections for Lumbosacral Radicular Pain." *Cochrane Database of Systematic Reviews* (4) (2020): CD013577. doi:10.1002/14651858.CD013577.

Sdrulla AD, Guan Y, and Raja SN. "Spinal Cord Stimulation: Clinical Efficacy and Potential Mechanisms." *Pain Practice* 18 (8) (November 2018): 1048–67. doi:10.1111/papr.12692. Epub: April 23, 2018. PMID: 29526043. PMCID: PMC6391880.

Traeger AC, Gilbert SE, Harris IA, and Maher CG. "Spinal Cord Stimulation for Low Back Pain." *Cochrane Database of Systematic Reviews* (3) (2023). doi:10.1002/14651858.CD014789.pub2.

Zhang W, Wang D, Li H, et al. "Mesenchymal Stem Cells Can Improve Discogenic Pain in Patients with Intervertebral Disc Degeneration: A Systematic Review and Meta-Analysis." *Frontiers in Bioengineering and Biotechnology* 11 (2023): 1155357. doi:10.3389/fbioe.2023.1155357.

Chapter 17

"Anesthesia Risks." Made for This Moment. Accessed October 19, 2025. https://www.asahq.org/madeforthismoment/anesthesia-101/types-of-anesthesia/anesthesia-risks/.

Bada ES, Gardner AC, Ahuja S, et al. "Lumbar Spine Fusion Surgery Versus Best Conservative Care for Patients with Severe, Persistent Low Back Pain." *Bone & Joint Open* 5 (7) (2024): 612–20. doi:10.1302/2633-1462.57.BJO-2023-0147.R1.

Chou R, Baisden J, Carragee EJ, Resnick DK, Shaffer WO, and Loeser JD. "Surgery for Low Back Pain: A Review of the Evidence for an American Pain Society Clinical Practice Guideline." *Spine* 34 (10) (2009): 1094–109. doi:10.1097/BRS.0b013e3181a105fc.

DePalma MG. "Red Flags of Low Back Pain." *JAAPA* 33 (8) (2020): 8–11. doi:10.1097/01.JAA.0000684112.91641.4c.

Etigunta SK, Liu AM, Gausper A, et al. "Long-Term Reoperation Rates After Single-Level Lumbar Discectomy: A Nationwide Cohort Study." *Spine* 50 (15) (2025): 1052–57. doi:10.1097/BRS.0000000000005328.

Fritzell P, Hägg O, Wessberg P, Nordwall A, and Swedish Lumbar Spine Study Group. "2001 Volvo Award Winner in Clinical Studies: Lumbar Fusion Versus Nonsurgical Treatment for Chronic Low Back Pain: A Multicenter Randomized Controlled Trial from the Swedish Lumbar Spine Study Group." *Spine* 26 (23) (2001): 2521–34. doi:10.1097/00007632-200112010-00002.

Giraldo JP, Williams GP, Lee JJ, Potts EA, and Uribe JS. "An Evidence-Based Review of the Current Surgical Treatments for Chronic Low-Back Pain: Rationale, Indications, and Novel Therapies." *Journal of Neurosurgery: Spine* 42 (4) (2025): 413–24. doi:10.3171/2024.9.SPINE24580.

Harris IA, Traeger A, Stanford R, Maher CG, and Buchbinder R. "Lumbar Spine Fusion: What Is the Evidence?" *Internal Medicine Journal* 48 (12) (2018): 1430–34. doi:10.1111/imj.14120.

Issa TZ, Ezeonu T, Sellig M, et al. "An Update in Complication Rates Associated with Anterior Lumbar Surgery: A Systematic Review and Meta-Analysis." *Global Spine Journal* 15 (2) (March 2025): 1419–34. doi:10.1177/21925682241279526. Epub: August 28, 2024. PMID: 39197439. PMCID: PMC11571399.

Jacobs WC, van der Gaag NA, Kruyt MC, et al. "Total Disc Replacement for Chronic Discogenic Low Back Pain: A Cochrane Review. *Spine* 38 (1) (2013): 24–36. doi:10.1097/BRS.0b013e3182741b21.

Ko S and Kwon J. "Does Discectomy Improve Low Back Pain as well as Radiating Pain in Patients with Lumbar Herniated Intervertebral Disc (HIVD)?" *Medicine* (Baltimore) 101 (1) (January 7, 2022): e27559. doi:10.1097/MD.0000000000027559. PMID: 35029870. PMCID: PMC8735808.

Lee MJ, Hacquebord J, Varshney A, et al. "Risk Factors for Medical Complication After Lumbar Spine Surgery: A Multivariate Analysis of 767 Patients." *Spine* 36 (21) (October 1, 2011): 1801–06. doi:10.1097/brs.0b013e318219d28d. PMID: 22046614. PMCID: PMC3711415.

Lewin AM, Fearnside M, Kuru R, et al. "Rates, Costs, Return to Work and Reoperation Following Spinal Surgery in a Workers' Compensation Cohort In New South Wales, 2010–2018: A Cohort Study Using Administrative Data." *BMC Health Services Research* 21 (1) (2021): 955. doi:10.1186/s12913-021-06900-8.

Lo YT, Lim-Watson M, Seo Y, et al. "Long-Term Opioid Prescriptions After Spine Surgery: A Meta-Analysis of Prevalence and Risk Factors." *World Neurosurgery* 141 (2020): e894–e920. doi:10.1016/j.wneu.2020.06.081.

"Mayo Clinic Q and A: Reduce Your Risk of Side Effects from Anesthesia by Liza Torborg." Mayo Clinic, September 6, 2019. https://newsnetwork.mayoclinic.org/discussion/mayo-clinic-q-and-a-reduce-your-risk-of-side-effects-from-anesthesia/.

Parker SL, Mendenhall SK, Godil SS, et al. "Incidence of Low Back Pain After Lumbar Discectomy for Herniated Disc and Its Effect on Patient-Reported Outcomes." *Clinical Orthopaedics and Related Research* 473 (6) (June 2015): 1988–99. doi:10.1007/s11999-015-4193-1. PMID: 25694267. PMCID: PMC4419014.

Chapter 18

Bair MJ, Matthias MS, Nyland KA, et al. "Barriers and Facilitators to Chronic Pain Self-Management: A Qualitative Study of Primary Care Patients with Comorbid Musculoskeletal Pain and Depression." *Pain Medicine* (Malden, MA) 10 (7) (2009): 1280–90. doi:10.1111/j.1526-4637.2009.00707.x.

Barlow J, Wright C, Sheasby J, Turner A, and Hainsworth J. "Self-Management Approaches for People with Chronic Conditions: A Review." *Patient Education and Counseling* 48 (2) (2002): 177–87. doi:10.1016/S0738-3991 (02)00032-0.

Bise CG, Schneider M, Freburger J, et al. "First Provider Seen for an Acute Episode of Low Back Pain Influences Subsequent Health Care Utilization." *Physical Therapy & Rehabilitation Journal* 103 (9) (2023): pzad067. doi:10.1093/ptj/pzad067.

Bourke MJ, Ferguson D, and Cooke M. "Patient Experiences of Self-Management for Chronic Low Back Pain: A Qualitative Study." *Physical Therapy & Rehabilitation Journal*. Published online March 30, 2022: pzac030. doi:10.1093/ptj/pzac030.

Elton D and Zhang M. "Low Back Pain Care Pathways—Is the Last Provider Seen More Important than the First: A Retrospective Cohort Study." *medRxiv*. Preprint posted online November 22, 2022. doi:10.1101/2022.10.27.22281624.

Frogner BK, Harwood K, Andrilla CHA, Schwartz M, and Pines JM. "Physical Therapy as the First Point of Care to Treat Low Back Pain: An Instrumental Variables Approach to Estimate Impact on Opioid Prescription, Health Care Utilization, and Costs." *Health Services Research* 53 (6) (2018): 4629–46. doi:10.1111/1475-6773.12984.

Hartvigsen J, Hancock MJ, Kongsted A, et al. "What Low Back Pain Is and Why We Need to Pay Attention." *Lancet* 391 (10137) (2018): 2356–67. doi:10.1016/S0140-6736(18)30480-X.

Herman PM, Edgington SE, Sorbero ME, Hurwitz EL, Goertz CM, and Coulter ID. "Visit Frequency and Outcomes for Patients Using Ongoing Chiropractic Care for Chronic Low Back and Neck Pain: An Observational Longitudinal Study." *Pain Physician* 24 (1) (2021): E61–E74.

Hutting N, Johnston V, Staal JB, and Heerkens YF. "Promoting the Use of Self-Management Strategies for People with Persistent Musculoskeletal Disorders: The Role of Physical Therapists. *Journal of Orthopaedic & Sports Physical Therapy* 49 (4) (2019): 212–15. doi:10.2519/jospt.2019.0605.

Kerr EA, Kullgren JT, and Saini SD. "Choosing Wisely: How to Fulfill the Promise in the Next 5 Years." *Health Affairs* (Millwood, VA) 36 (11) (2017): 2012–18. doi:10.1377/hlthaff.2017.0953.

Saragiotto BT, Maher CG, Traeger AC, Li Q, and McAuley JH. "Dispelling the Myth That Chronic Pain Is Unresponsive to Treatment." *British Journal of Sports Medicine* 51 (13) (2017): 986–88. doi:10.1136/bjsports-2016-096821.

Wiles LK, Hibbert PD, Stephens JH, et al. "What Constitutes 'Appropriate Care' for Low Back Pain? Point-of-Care Clinical Indicators from Guideline Evidence and Experts (the STANDING

Collaboration Project)." *Spine*. Published online November 22, 2021. doi:10.1097/BRS.0000000000004274.

Zadro J, O'Keeffe M, and Maher C. "Do Physical Therapists Follow Evidence-Based Guidelines When Managing Musculoskeletal Conditions? Systematic Review." *BMJ Open* 9 (10) (2019): e032329. doi:10.1136/bmjopen-2019-032329.

Chapter 21

Belavy DL, Tagliaferri SD, Buntine P, et al. "Reducing Low-Value Imaging for Low Back Pain: Systematic Review with Meta-Analysis." *Journal of Orthopaedic & Sports Physical Therapy* 52 (4) (2022): 175–91. doi:10.2519/jospt.2022.10731.

Buchbinder R, Underwood M, Hartvigsen J, and Maher CG. "The Lancet Series Call to Action to Reduce Low Value Care for Low Back Pain: An Update." *Pain* 161 (Suppl 1) (1) (2020): S57–S64. doi:10.1097/j.pain.0000000000001869.

"Claims Denials and Appeals in ACA Marketplace Plans in 2023." KFF, January 27, 2025. https://www.kff.org/private-insurance/claims-denials-and-appeals-in-aca-marketplace-plans-in-2023/.

Darlow B and O'Sullivan PB. "Why Are Back Pain Guidelines Left on the Sidelines? Three Myths Appear to be Guiding Management of Back Pain in Sport." *British Journal of Sports Medicine* 50 (21) (2016): 1294–95. doi:10.1136/bjsports-2016-096312.

Fritz JM, Cleland JA, and Brennan GP. "Does Adherence to the Guideline Recommendation for Active Treatments Improve the Quality of Care for Patients with Acute Low Back Pain Delivered by Physical Therapists?" *Medical Care* 45 (10) (2007): 973–80. doi:10.1097/MLR.0b013e318070c6cd.

Goertz CM and George SZ. "Insurer Coverage of Nonpharmacological Treatments for Low Back Pain—Time for a Change." *JAMA Network Open* 1 (6) (2018): e183037. doi:10.1001/jamanetworkopen.2018.3037.

Hartvigsen J, Kamper SJ, and French SD. "Low-Value Care in Musculoskeletal Health Care: Is There a Way Forward?" *Pain Practice* 22 (Suppl 2) (2022): 65–70. doi:10.1111/papr.13142.

Heyward J, Jones CM, Compton WM, et al. "Coverage of Nonpharmacologic Treatments for Low Back Pain Among US Public and Private Insurers." *JAMA Network Open* 1 (6) (2018): e183044. doi:10.1001/jamanetworkopen.2018.3044.

Hong AS, Ross-Degnan D, Zhang F, and Wharam JF. "Small Decline in Low-Value Back Imaging Associated with the 'Choosing Wisely' Campaign, 2012–14." *Health Affairs* (Project HOPE) 36 (4) (2017): 671–79. doi:10.1377/hlthaff.2016.1263.

Lin I, Wiles L, Waller R, et al. "What Does Best Practice Care for Musculoskeletal Pain Look Like? Eleven Consistent Recommendations from High-Quality Clinical Practice Guidelines: Systematic Review." *British Journal of Sports Medicine* 54 (2) (2020): 79–86. doi:10.1136/bjsports-2018-099878.

Radomski TR, Zhao X, Lovelace EZ, et al. "Use and Cost of Low-Value Health Services Delivered or Paid for by the Veterans Health Administration." *JAMA Internal Medicine* 182 (8) (2022): 832–39. doi:10.1001/jamainternmed.2022.2482.

Viana da Silva P, Kamper SJ, Robson E, et al. "'Myths and Facts' Education Is Comparable to 'Facts Only' for Recall of Back Pain Information but May Improve Fear-Avoidance Beliefs: An Embedded Randomized Trial." *Journal of Orthopaedic & Sports Physical Therapy*. Published online July 8, 2022: 1–29. doi:10.2519/jospt.2022.10989.

Zadro J, O'Keeffe M, and Maher C. "Do Physical Therapists Follow Evidence-Based Guidelines When Managing Musculoskeletal Conditions? Systematic Review." *BMJ Open* 9 (10) (2019): e032329. doi:10.1136/bmjopen-2019-032329.

Chapter 22

Bailly F, Trouvin AP, Bercier S, et al. "Clinical Guidelines and Care Pathway for Management of Low Back Pain with or Without Radicular Pain." *Joint Bone Spine* 88 (6) (2021): 105227. doi:10.1016/j.jbspin.2021.105227.

Buelt A, McCall S, and Coster J. "Management of Low Back Pain: Guidelines from the VHA/DoD." *American Family Physician* 107 (4) (2023): 435–37.

Dowell D, Ragan KR, Jones CM, et al. "CDC Clinical Practice Guideline for Prescribing Opioids for Pain—United States, 2022." *MMWR* 71 (3) (2022): 1-95. doi:10.15585/mmwr.rr7103a1.

Fritz JM, Cleland JA, and Brennan GP. "Does Adherence to the Guideline Recommendation for Active Treatments Improve the Quality of Care for Patients with Acute Low Back Pain Delivered by Physical Therapists?" *Medical Care* 45 (10) (2007): 973–80. doi:10.1097/MLR.0b013e318070c6cd.

George SZ, Fritz JM, Silfies SP, et al. "Interventions for the Management of Acute and Chronic Low Back Pain: Revision 2021." *Journal of Orthopaedic & Sports Physical Therapy* 51 (11) (2021): CPG1–CPG60. doi:10.2519/jospt.2021.0304.

Globe G, Farabaugh RJ, Hawk C, et al. "Clinical Practice Guideline: Chiropractic Care for Low Back Pain." *Journal of Manipulative and Physiological Therapeutics* 39 (1) (2016): 1–22. doi:10.1016/j.jmpt.2015.10.006.

National Guideline Centre (UK). *Low Back Pain and Sciatica in Over 16s: Assessment and Management.* London: National Institute for Health and Care Excellence (UK), 2016. http://www.ncbi.nlm.nih.gov/books/NBK401577/.

Qaseem A, Wilt TJ, McLean RM, Forciea MA, and Clinical Guidelines Committee of the American College of Physicians. "Noninvasive Treatments for Acute, Subacute, and Chronic Low Back Pain: A Clinical Practice Guideline from the American College of Physicians." *Annals of Internal Medicine* 166 (7) (2017): 514–30. doi:10.7326/M16-2367.

"WHO Guideline for Non-Surgical Management of Chronic Primary Low Back Pain in Adults in Primary and Community Care Settings." World Health Organization. Accessed December 15, 2023. https://www.who.int/publications-detail-redirect/9789240081789.

Index

A

B

C

D

E

F

G

H

I

J

K

L

R

S

T

X

Y

Z

About the Author

Christine Goertz, DC, PhD, is a professor in musculoskeletal research and vice chair for implementation of spine health innovations in the Department of Orthopaedic Surgery at Duke University School of Medicine, where she spearheaded the Duke Spine Health Program. She is also an adjunct professor in the Department of Epidemiology at the University of Iowa College of Public Health. A leading voice in nondrug treatment for spine-related disorders, Dr. Goertz directs interdisciplinary research teams focused on the intersection of rigorous research, real-world care and health policy. Dr. Goertz has coauthored more than 150 scientific papers, been cited over 7,000 times and secured nearly $45 million in federal funding as a principal investigator. She was ranked among the top ten NIH-funded investigators in orthopedics by the Blue Ridge Institute for Medical Research in 2022, 2023, and 2024. Dr. Goertz earned her doctor of chiropractic degree from Northwestern Health Sciences University and her PhD in health services research, policy, and administration from the University of Minnesota School of Public Health.